DEMENTIA and YOU

Care, Protection and Reducing the Risk

Dr. Ross M. Colquhoun

ISBN: 150787927X
ISBN 13: 9781507879276
Library of Congress Control Number: **XXXXX (If applicable)**
LCCN Imprint Name: **City and State (If applicable)**

This book is dedicated to the memory of my mother, Daphne Ross Colquhoun.

Contents

Forward

The complex challenge of the rising epidemic of dementia in Australia is one I face every day as a general medical practitioner. This challenge is only beginning to be understood by our communities.

Dr. Ross Colquhoun's book offers a multifaceted analysis of the issues raised by dementia and explores the solutions to these. This book covers a lot of ground, from basic medical issues through to psychosocial, legal, and family concerns. This is not just an academic book, but offers real support and direction for those working with people with dementia in a personal or professional capacity.

Dr. Colquhoun offers a blend of good scientific research and heartwarming experience of working with those with dementia and their families. For anyone trying to understand what dementia is through to those who need guidance in their daily involvement with those with dementia, this book is essential reading.

Dr. David Hunt

General Practitioner

Chairman, Teen Challenge, Queensland

It is a privilege to write a forward to this book, a second edition of Ross's book dealing with dementia. Ross is a highly qualified health scientist with a doctorate degree. He is a man who really has wanted and wants to "change the world" for those struggling with personal, family, and social issues, for example, dementia, aging, and drug addiction.

Now through this book, he is enlightening us all about the personal and social problem of dementia we face with an aging population. Dementia and related conditions will need to be addressed by families, society, and governments as a matter of urgency.

Ross outlines his approach to a better, empathetic, and more cost-effective way of handling this issue that affects us all. This is the Dr. Ross Colquhoun I have had the honor of knowing and working with. It is a must-read for all.

Dr. Barry Landa

General Practitioner and Family Physician

Preface to the Second Edition

I'm still not sure writing this new book on dementia will convince my children to be kind to me if or when I succumb to dementia. I hope they at least read it and ponder on what was going through my mind as I wrote it. More importantly they will find in this new edition a change in perspective and a change in my view of dementia and what can be done to prevent it. The first book reflected much of the sense of doom and gloom around dementia, as reflected in the research of the time. I feared I would succumb just as my mother had.

OUT OF ADVERSITY CAME A HAPPIER DISPOSITION.

This new book is far more optimistic and hopeful. This is not just wishful thinking but arises from new evidence from long-term studies and new discoveries about the causes and prevention of chronic disease, including dementia.

I completed the first version of this book when I was fifty-eight and I took some comfort from the fact I had been able to finish it. I also mentioned, again without much conviction, that I took some comfort from the belief that doing this type of activity was meant to protect me from getting dementia. I am now sixty-four, and much has changed. I am now working in China teaching at a University. This fulfills a life-long dream. Most significantly I was nearly killed in a motorcycle accident.

Someone at work had given me a plaque saying "Adventure Before Dementia." All very amusing: I bought a Harley and set off, leather outfit, badges, and all, with a "gang" of grisly-looking men who were mostly older than I. No one said premature death might also be a consequence of this adventure. Well, they did say I was stupid, but as they also said, "Go for it; you won't be here forever."

I SLOWLY RECOVERED AND BECAME MORE CONSCIOUS OF MY HEALTH

Having ended up underneath a semitrailer with broken vertebrae, broken ribs, nerve damage, knee and ankle injuries, and head injuries, I hung up the boots and helmet and changed my life direction. While I slowly recovered, I also became more conscious of my health, did more research, and had more time to ponder on the sort of life I wanted. I think this book reflects that change. Out of adversity came an altogether more positive perspective and happier disposition. And the opportunity to go to China!

However, my interest in the subject of dementia started with my mother. While I have academic qualifications in psychology, neuroscience and health science I recall at the time of my mother's illness, as a family, we struggled to understand what was happening, the extent of the burden my father carried and what we could do. My original aim was to write a book that accurately reflected the reality of dementia, but also a book anyone could pick up and easily read and understand.

> SHE TOLD OF HOW ONE PARTNER AFTER ANOTHER DESERTED HER.

Since publication of the first edition, 6 years ago now, I have regularly talked to seniors groups. The feedback from the first edition confirmed I had to a large extent succeeded. However, there was a lot more that people wanted to know. Mainly questions about prevention were repeatedly asked. This book sets out to answer those questions and many others that arose during this time. And it neatly tied in with the changed priorities in my life.

My mother was a very smart woman, although most of her productive years were taken up devotedly caring for me and my brother and sister. It was not until her later years, after she was well into her fifties, as a result of a near-fatal car accident, she hung up her beloved golf clubs, and she started playing contract bridge. Within a short time, she had become a district master, a state master, and then a national master of this game. It seems it requires remarkable feats of memory to get to this level. Players sought her out as their partner to play in competitions in the hope she would carry them upward. I've heard there are many dedicated players who spend their lives and their money going to bridge congresses to play the game all over the world and never make district master!

> ## SHE DIDN'T HAVE MUCH TIME FOR THOSE WHO SHE THOUGHT WERE FOOLS

Some twenty years later, I can vividly see an image of my mother weeping inconsolably as she told of one partner after another deserting her and some even insulting her. This was the start of her battle with dementia, although she didn't understand what was happening then; and soon, so it seemed, she was not really able to remember much at all. She would often start to prepare her lunch only a short time after finishing a hearty meal. She would forget we had seen her the week before, and she would think my daughter was her daughter.

I remember going with her to the local aged-care assessment team to see if we could get some help for her and my father around their house. She didn't have much time for those who she thought were fools, and even then she would castigate those she thought were rude or not paying attention. Anyway, we were grateful for the help, as going to her home was difficult for some of us as she didn't seem to see the dirt covering most things or the food on a "new" dress she would don for some outing.

> WE WERE SAVED FROM MAKING MANY DECISIONS AS MY FATHER DUTIFULLY CARED FOR HER.

Above all I remember her delight at seeing the grandchildren, even though after a little while their antics would wear on her patience. She also enjoyed her whiskey or sherry in the evening, and for some years, despite the short-term memory loss, she seemed to be able to knock off cryptic crosswords in no time. I think we were saved from making the sorts of decisions families are often faced with as my father dutifully cared for her and shielded her from danger and embarrassment until she died quietly of pneumonia when she was eighty-four.

While my father got a bit obsessive about things, he never really stopped functioning at a pretty high level until he passed on a year later, suffering from grief and sadness after the loss of his partner of over fifty years. I believe his time caring for my mother gave him a real sense of purpose, even though he would often chide her for her forgetfulness. Without her he had nothing left to do.

Even though my mother could not escape the clutches of dementia, what a rich and satisfying life my parents had.

I FEEL MORE OPTIMISTIC ABOUT LIVING A WELL AND FULFILLING LIFE

As they grew older, both of them would spend time telling us about their lives as children, growing up in an era of horses and carts, dunnymen collecting the cans and ice being delivered by these means, seeing the first cars on the streets, listening to crackling radios, and of course, their years in the army.

My father spent time in North Africa, Greece, and then the Kokoda Trail, as well as the war in the Pacific, where he won a Military Cross for bravery. My mother was posted to Darwin as a nurse, and she told stories of the Japanese bombing of the city. She rose to the rank of Major, much to my father's displeasure as he only became a Captain! And then they told stories together of their time with the occupation forces in Japan, where they met.

Indeed, they were the lucky members of their generation, having escaped an early death despite the dangers of childbirth, infectious disease, the war, and the cancers and heart disease that took many of their friends.

As I ponder on their lives and mine, it is with deep gratitude I remember the chances they gave me to live a full and privileged life.

> I FEEL HEALTHIER TODAY HAVING MADE CHANGES TO THE WAY I CARE FOR MYSELF.

In the first edition of this book, I hoped I would live for some years yet to see my grandchildren grow to be young adults, but I felt it was likely I would suffer from dementia. There was, however, one aspect of my mother's life I did not mention, as it seemed almost irrelevant: my mother was a smoker from the time she joined the army until she passed away. We now know smoking is a major cause of oxidative stress, and we now know that this is a major cause of cell dysfunction and chronic disease. I wondered what impact sixty years of inhaling cigarette smoke had on her cardiovascular system and eventual dementia. I then started to read further afield and to understand that many of the diseases that take so much enjoyment from our later years are preventable.

Hence, this new book is much more than an account of dementia to promote discussion and an understanding about how to cope with it; it is primarily a declaration that we can do much to control our destiny, as lifestyle change can make a profound difference.

> ### WE DON'T HAVE TO LIVE WITH PAIN AND DISABILITY.

I now feel much healthier today, as I have made changes to improve the way I eat and exercise, take vitamins and antioxidants, reduce stress, and take better care of myself.

Consequently I feel more optimistic about living a well and fulfilling life for some years yet. And I want to share that belief with my fellow baby boomers and our children and grandchildren. I believe we can make choices to minimize pain, suffering mental failure and disability and the indignity that comes with it. Chronic disease, including dementia, is preventable, but it lies with us to act to change the way we choose to live.

Chapter 1

About Dementia

Aging and illness are subjects we would rather not think about, let alone talk about, especially when the early signs indicate something serious like dementia or Alzheimer's disease is happening to you or your loved ones. To many, dementia means loss of memory, the inability to manage affairs, and loss of dignity. A healthy and well-functioning mind is most important and most essential to experiencing and expressing joy, engaging in socialization and relationships, reminiscing about times gone by, and being creative.

> NOT THAT LONG AGO, PEOPLE MOSTLY DIED OF ILLNESSES OTHER THAN DEMENTIA.

Dementia means the loss of humanity and self-awareness. Eventually it will lead to death, and there is nothing we can do about it as there is no cure as yet.

However, like many other chronic diseases, new evidence indicates that dementia is preventable. The scientific opinion now leans toward the idea that the cause of all dementias is related to oxidative stress leading to cell dysfunction and cardiovascular disease, such as clogged arteries, causing decreased blood flow and circulation of nutrients and oxygen to the brain. When these systems fail, cells are damaged and die, and disease processes are not able to be defended against. This insight suggests that things like diet, exercise, avoiding pollutants like smog and smoking, and lack of optimal nutrition can be modified to prevent dementia by making lifestyle changes. But this has to happen at an early stage, as many brain cells are dead or dying by the time dementia is diagnosed.

> I WAS CONCERNED ABOUT BEING A BURDEN ON MY
> CHILDREN.

One of the original aims of this book was to provide information to those aged between forty-six and sixty-six who were concerned they might be showing signs of dementia or else believed they might be at risk: the baby-boomer generation. You will find that many of your questions will be answered. It may even be helpful for those who are younger and have worries about not thinking clearly or becoming forgetful. Most importantly, if you are worried, this book may convince you to seek early assessment. You can then determine just what is going on, what will happen in the future, and what you can do now while you can still make clear decisions for yourself.

Hopefully you will understand that, like cancer, the earlier you know what is happening, the earlier you can take preventive action and get help to relieve symptoms and maximize your independence and quality of life. Most importantly it might motivate you to make changes in your lifestyle to reduce the risk of getting not only dementia, but also other chronic diseases like heart disease, diabetes, arthritis, cancer, and respiratory diseases.

I HOPE MY CONCERNS ARE YOUR CONCERNS

When I referred to "our generation" in the book, I was mainly talking about people in their fifties or sixties. In other words I was talking about my generation and my misgivings about losing my faculties and becoming reliant on my children or strangers to help me function. And about being a burden on them, but also about not being abandoned. It also served to make me examine my attitude to the way I live so it is less likely I will have to rely on them.

Like many of us, I fear dementia, and I wanted to know what I could do about it. I hoped that my concerns were your concerns, and we could both learn from this book. Even more, I wanted my children to read it so they would know what to do with me when I was grumpy (or more grumpy), forgot their birthdays, or did not recognize them anymore—

as well as recognize when it was unsafe for me to be left alone for too long. And I wanted them to think about the day these diseases might affect them and the changes they might make to their lifestyle and the environment to reduce the risk of that happening to them and their children.

However, this book is also designed to answer questions and provide helpful information for those who have loved ones they believe are suffering from dementia, even if it has not been diagnosed. That is the next generation, the children and grandchildren who will have to cope with this problem in the next few years.

DEMENTIA IS FREQUENTLY MISDIAGNOSED.

It can also be helpful for those, whose parents are well into the latter years, and for husbands and wives of those who may already be showing signs of dementia or have been diagnosed as having dementia. Caring for someone with dementia can be very stressful. I hope this book can provide some guidance.

Some of the greatest problems with dementia are that many people are never diagnosed and are not treated, as well as the frequency of misdiagnosis and inappropriate treatment. This book will give you some idea of what to expect when faced with the reality of dementia and what you can do to ensure the best outcome for you or your loved one. It will also help you as a caregiver to protect your own welfare, to ensure that you don't become exhausted and resentful. This is only possible when early diagnosis is made and early treatment is implemented.

Chapters 4 and 5 describe the symptoms of dementia and what to expect, while Chapter 6 is devoted to providing some suggestions to help you communicate effectively so the reality of dementia can be discussed openly.

NOT KNOWING CAN MAKE THINGS WORSE.

Chapter 7 is mainly for caregivers and tackles the sense of grief and loss they are faced with while caring for a loved one with dementia. In chapter 8 I have spent some time talking about respectful and effective communication that is designed to build rapport and to include, as much as possible, the person with dementia in the whole assessment and treatment-planning process. It can then be possible to devise strategies to support and improve the quality of life and dignity of you or the person you are concerned about, taking into account preferences and plans for the future. The suggestions are practical ones for improving functioning, not just dwelling on the disease or the symptoms. Most importantly I have written new sections (chapters 9 and 10) that discuss strategies to reduce the risk and impact of dementia, and other chronic diseases, through changes in lifestyle and caring strategies.

I have also written a section on how professionals can help, not just with assessment, but also with treatment planning (chapter 11); and another section (chapter 12) on finding the right solution when people can no longer cope on their own. Chapter 13 discusses quality of life for the person with advanced dementia and in chapter 14 what to do about the legal issues that can arise.

EVERYONE BENEFITS FROM A HEALTHY LIFESTYLE.

Dementia can be viewed with fear and uncertainty, or it can be understood. Preventative strategies and treatments can then be developed as soon as we know what is happening in order to maintain a good quality of life as long as possible. While we are living longer, there is an increasing tendency to spend more time with declining health. Leaving it alone can make matters worse—and "leaving it alone" includes not treating other problems that can look like dementia or make the symptoms worse. Most importantly I suggest you be guided in your decisions by the person with dementia. Find out what they want, what preparations you can make for his or her care, and how to protect his or her interests before it is too late.

However, this new book offers much more. New research shows that the incidence of dementia will not be as high as predicted, that chronic disease is preventable, and that lifestyle change is the most important factor in prevention. While acknowledging the reality of dementia, this new book is also about hope and about taking control of our lives.

DEMENTIA WILL SOON BE THE BIGGEST CAUSE OF DEATH.

We know that, like cancer, dementia has its beginnings many years before it is diagnosed. The presence of cancer is often foreshadowed by precancerous polyps, lesions, and ill-formed cells that eventually result in cancer. So also dementia has its origins in the damage to individual cells that fail to reproduce properly, and it is thought to begin many years before it becomes apparent.

It all starts with maintaining a healthy heart and blood circulation system and, most importantly, a healthy protective or immune system. Modern medicine intervenes when diseases become apparent, often when it is too late to make any significant difference. Instead of waiting for the worst to happen, we can adapt strategies to minimize damage, aid in the repair of damaged cells, and maximize the regeneration of healthy cells. This strategy is based on the fact that optimal nourishment and protection from oxidative stress (free radicals) can allow the body to heal itself. As a consequence this book has relevance to readers of all ages who would like to examine the benefits of making healthy lifestyle choices.

LIFESTYLE CHANGES CAN MAKE A DIFFERENCE

Choices to strengthen the body's immune system to protect against cell damage and to prevent disease should be made as early as possible. As mentioned, chapter 9 will look at exercise, diet, and nutritional supplements and the evidence that these lifestyle changes can make a difference.

In the next part of the book, in chapters 2 and 3 , I want to put dementia into context. The next chapter will answer some questions about why it has now emerged as a major health problem and why so many of us will contract the disease.

Chapter 2

Dementia: what is it and why we are at risk now?

A short while ago, cancer was viewed in the same way as dementia is now: a death sentence, as there was no cure and no hope. And it was not that long ago that cancer was rare and people mostly died of other illnesses, like pneumonia, tuberculosis, polio, and other infectious diseases. But then people often only lived until their fifties, and an old person was one who lived beyond his or her sixties.

> ALZHEIMER'S DISEASE AND VASCULAR DEMENTIA ARE COMMON TYPES OF DEMENTIA.

Antibiotics and other medical advances meant that people were much less likely to die of infectious diseases. Diseases like heart disease, stroke, and, of course, cancer caused fear and apprehension because they were going to get us. But then again, we were living much longer, and people expected to live until they were seventy at least.

It will not be many years before dementia will be the biggest cause of death rather than heart disease, stroke, and cancer, and it is simply that modern science has meant we can often escape the clutches of these other diseases.

Studies from the United States show that from 2000 to 2006, Alzheimer's disease deaths increased 46.1 percent, while other causes of death decreased. Investments in research and new treatments for other diseases have resulted in declines in deaths for some of these diseases. For example, during this same period, heart disease deaths decreased by 11.1 percent and stroke by 18.2 percent. Remarkably, since 1950 when America was ranked seventh in the world in terms of life expectancy and despite ever-increasing budgets for health, by 2009 it was ranked twenty-seventh.

ANYONE OVER SIXTY IS AT RISK OF DEMENTIA.

As we live longer, waiting for us are new diseases, and dementia is the most likely and the most feared.

For anyone over sixty, there is a chance of developing a degenerative disease of the brain. There are many afflictions of this type that develop in old age, however, the one that is most well known is dementia: Sometimes called senile dementia or Alzheimer's disease, the most common type.

Dementia is defined as an acquired syndrome of decline in memory and at least one other mental capacity, such as language, orientation, or planning and thinking, sufficient to interfere with social or occupational functioning in an alert person. "Mild cognitive impairment" is a more mild condition not associated with functional impairment that sometimes progresses to dementia. And, of course, we all tend to become forgetful and vague as a condition of aging.

Between 60 and 70 percent of individuals with dementia are thought to have Alzheimer's disease; about 20 to 30 percent have either vascular dementia or a combination of vascular dementia and Alzheimer's disease.

AGE IS THE STRONGEST RISK FACTOR FOR DEMENTIA.

The disease causes a high burden of suffering for people with dementia and their families. For those with dementia, it increases dependency and complicates other medical conditions, and it can lead to anxiety and depression. For families it is a stressful time not knowing what is happening or what to do and how to create the time needed to care for loved ones.

Because of the aging population and declining birthrate, dementias like Alzheimer's disease are quickly becoming a major health problem. They will soon overtake rates for depression, and in a few years, they will be the single greatest cause of death. While only some five thousand people in Australia under sixty are diagnosed with

Alzheimer's, one in four people over eighty will suffer and die from the disease.

Age is the strongest risk factor for dementia: 3 to 11 percent of people older than sixty-five and 25 to 47 percent of those older than eighty-five have dementia. It is estimated that the proportion of the population aged over sixty-five with the disease will soon double from the present 13 percent. First-degree relatives of patients with Alzheimer's disease have a cumulative lifetime risk of 39 percent, approximately twice the risk of Alzheimer's disease in the general population. In other words we can inherit the disease, although this is only one factor and not a major one.

PHYSICAL EXERCISE AND DIET CAN TO HELP.

Cardiovascular risk factors, such as high blood pressure (hypertension), are more highly associated with an increased risk of both Alzheimer's disease and vascular dementia.

There is now ample evidence to indicate cardiovascular risk factors are linked to degenerative processes preceding cognitive decline in dementia, as well as mild cognitive impairment (MCI). Decreased blood flow to the brain negatively affects protein synthesis, which is necessary for memory and learning, and may eventually lead to brain cell injury and death. Since the mid-1990s, imaging techniques have shown this link. Studies using imaging techniques showed that a decline in nutrients and oxygen to the brain increased with severity of dementia, and the severity of blood flow to the brain corresponded with the severity of the disease. Significant links were found between language and blood flow to the language centers of the brain and visuospatial abilities and blood flow.

SOME DEMENTIAS ARE MORE TREATABLE THAN OTHERS.

Irrespective of other factors that may or may not be related to the breakdown of thinking ability, imaging studies show that failures of adequate blood flow may lead to cognitive decline and gradual and progressive brain-cell death. Amazingly, the flow of nutrients and oxygen to the brain is finely tuned and regulated to meet the demands of the brain according to the cognitive activity it is engaged in. These processes are complicated and highly sensitive to deficits in the nutrients the brain needs to function well.

Hence, the link between cardiovascular dysfunction and dementia is well established. However, it is still not clear whether cardiovascular dysfunction is common to all these different types of dementia and to what extent. The fact is that several risk factors, such as cardiovascular disease, high blood pressure, diabetes, and obesity, enhance the rate of cognitive decline and increase the risk of dementia and Alzheimer's disease in particular. Also implicated are oxidative stress and nutrient deficiencies, all of which may be modifiable with lifestyle changes.

DEMENTIA IS NOT A NORMAL PART OF AGING.

Often associated with dementia is the loss of memory; however, there are different types of dementia, and not all show early memory failure. Sometimes the onset is marked by changes in mood, movement, or behavior, and often onset is so gradual we find it hard to connect this with a disease like dementia. Moreover, there are other reasons people start to forget things. These include the normal aging process, depression, stress, hormone and vitamin deficiencies, and physical ailments like brain tumors and infections; and all these can be happening separately or together, only making it even more confusing.

While many dementias are difficult to treat, or even to delay the onset or slow the progress of, some dementias respond to treatment, and other problems resulting in dementia-type symptoms can be treated. There are many types of dementia, and some are more treatable than others. In the meantime researchers are busy finding new treatments that will make a real difference.

More importantly we now have evidence that physical exercise, social activity, diet and nutrition, and an active mind prevent dementia or, at least, delay the onset for those at risk. One study even suggests that moderate alcohol use and gardening might guard against getting dementia. Certainly being overweight, having high blood pressure, and reduction in lung capacity (smoking, respiratory disease) are associated with increased risk. On the other hand, keeping the brain active, like learning a foreign language, is believed to protect against dementia.

MANY COUNTRIES ARE EXPERIENCING CHANGE.

Depression and worry are also related to increased risk of dementia. A whole range of treatments exists for risky behavior like overeating or smoking and psychological problems like depression and anxiety, including psychotherapy and medication.

Until recently it was thought that only one in twenty people will develop dementia in their sixties. However, by the time they reach their eighties, this can become as high as one in three, and 30 percent of people over ninety have dementia. In Australia there are now some 315,000 people who are sufferers; however, in thirty-five years' time, this is predicted to be over 1,000,000. Presently there are 1,300 new cases of dementia diagnosed each week. However, based on experience, in fifteen years' time, it is estimated that there will be 3,600 and in thirty-five years some 7,400 new cases each week. This trend is common to most advanced Western countries, and while it is a very disturbing process for both those with dementia and their families, it threatens to be a major burden to health systems and economies worldwide.

RESEARCH SHOWS CHANGING RATES OF DEMENTIA.

In England, with a population of 50 million, 16 percent of the population is over sixty-five, and there are estimated to be 700,000 with dementia, and this is likely to grow to over 1.5 million in thirty years. The cost to the health budget is 17 billion pounds—more than the cost of cancer, stroke, and heart disease combined. In Japan, 22.2 percent, or 28.3 million people, are over sixty-five, with 2.3 million people with dementia.

In 2002 in the United States, it was estimated that a total of 3.8 million individuals had dementia, and just over 2.5 million had Alzheimer's disease. Recently the Alzheimer's Association estimated there are now 5 million Americans with Alzheimer's disease. It is the sixth-leading cause of death in the United States and the fifth-leading cause of death in those aged sixty-five and older. More recently it was suggested that as many as 6.8 million people in the United States have dementia, and at least 1.8 million of those are severely affected.

With increasing numbers of older adults, Asian nations and their governments are faced with various social and economic issues for both the family and state.

CAREGIVER ISSUES ARE A MAJOR CONCERN.

Many countries are experiencing dramatic changes in the physical and social environment brought about by economic development. Urbanization, industrialization, migration, and most recently, globalization are causing changes in families and the intergenerational support of elderly people. A World Bank report showed that informal support systems are breaking down in countries like China. Caregiver issues are of major concern, as old age often brings with it dependency and impaired functioning, and everywhere people and governments are concerned about the provision of care for the growing number and proportion of aged. The challenge for public policy is to assess the viability of family support systems and to devise programs that will be supportive or complementary.

As populations across the world age and diagnosis rates increase, dementia is predicted to become more common and impact more lives. Although it is common in very elderly individuals, it is not considered a normal part of the aging process. Many people live into their nineties and even hundreds without any signs of dementia.

WE ARE LUCKY BECAUSE WE WILL LIVE LONGER

The next chapter is about our generation: the lucky generation. How can that be after all the bad news about dementia? How can this be right, when our generation is the one that will have to deal with this dreadful disease in numbers unheard-of in the past? If dementia is such a problem—incurable, degrading, with a loss of respect, dignity, independence, and control, confinement to a nursing home, and certain death—how can we be the lucky generation? We are lucky because on average we will live longer than any other generation before us and maybe even longer than future generations. More so, as it seems the predictions about rates of dementia were overestimated and the incidence of dementia among baby boomers will not be as high. In the next chapter I will talk about the latest research indicating changes in the rates of dementia in the coming years.

Chapter 3

The Lucky Generation

It seems that the generation born between 1945 and 1965 will live longer than any previous generation. And it may be the only future generation to do so. It seems the next generation will kill themselves off due to preventable lifestyle disease like heart disease, stroke, cancer, and diabetes—the same diseases many of the Lucky Generation escaped.

> THE NEXT GENERATION MAY NOT LIVE AS LONG.

Why? Obesity, a sedentary lifestyle, increased use of chemicals in food, and pollution. Ironically many will also die from infectious diseases in numbers unheard-of for over a century. Infections will be caused by new super-bugs— bacteria that have changed into forms our antibiotics cannot kill because of the overuse of these drugs and because we feed them to the animals we eat.

We are lucky because on average we have been able to survive longer than any humans before and perhaps after us. Not only are we able to survive longer; we do it in better health, but also we benefit from a lifestyle that has not yet become too crowded or frantic, too competitive or conflictual. Space will become a luxury and resources more scarce, and the disparity between rich and poor will increase as the population rapidly increases. The next generations will look back at this time and envy a world that is only known through the pages of a history textbook...or an online version of history. The gift of life we have been given is a super-serve.

WE HAVE LEARNED HOW OUR BRAIN WORKS

It is also a time when we have rapidly progressed in our understanding of our health and the cause of chronic disease and the role of lifestyle, exercise, diet, and supplements. We also have learned a great deal about our brain and how it works and the building blocks of life: the human genome.

The brain is an incredibly complex organism that enables us to be aware of our existence; it allows us to reflect on who we are and what we might be, and it is the source of our individuality. The brain contains 10 billion nerve cells, and it controls all our mental functions, including hunger, thirst, and sleep, and our capacity to remember and think. The impact of dementia diminishes these fundamental faculties. Scientists can now closely examine nerve cells and the connections among them and trace the instantaneously sent signals that control our every thought and movement and our very being. While we are lucky to have been born in a time of plenty, it behooves us to take precious care of this amazing gift. It is our capacity to make choices for our own and our planet's welfare that is the greatest of these gifts.

WE ARE NOT DESTINED TO GET DEMENTIA.

The brain is like the body's computer system. We retrieve a vast amount of information from the environment through our senses of touch, taste, smell, sight, and hearing. The brain translates the signals, amplifies the content, and makes meaning of it; it filters the information and sorts and stores it. The brain then provides that data in an accessible form for us to act on that information. The nervous system acts as an intricate and high-speed signaling circuit that relays the messages from the external and internal world to the brain and sends out signals to allow us to react appropriately. There are two parts to the nervous system: the brain and the spinal column and the peripheral connecting fibers that control automatic function and voluntary movement.

How intelligent we are is not a product of the size of the brain, as we once thought. It is entirely related to the number and quality of connections among the nerve cells.

Of great importance to our understanding of our brains and our capacity to alter our destiny is the new field of epigenetics. When the human genome was deciphered and mapped, it was discovered that we only had some 25,000 active genes, where we expected to find 100,000 or more.

The millions of leftover pieces of DNA were thought to be mere "junk" DNA that served no purpose. But how could it be that only 25,000 genes could determine our features, our personality, and our uniqueness?

EVERY PERSON CAN ALTER HIS OR HER DESTINY

It is now thought that all these junk DNA are dormant or "silent," ready to make or "express" proteins in response to the environment. In other words, every person can alter his or her destiny. Changes in gene expression relate to what we are exposed to and how we react, including what we eat, what stress we expose ourselves to, and how healthy we maintain our bodies and minds. And incredibly, it seems we might pass these changes on to our offspring!

So it seems we are not destined to succumb to dementia and that we can actively work at preventing it or delaying it, just as we can with diabetes or heart disease. The latest research suggests that the projections of the numbers who will get dementia may be wrong. It seems that due to our healthy diet, reduced smoking rates and pollution, education, stimulating work roles, and constant interaction with the outside world through multimedia far fewer than had been predicted will get dementia.

Smoking, stress (as excessive release of corticosteroids may have neurotoxic effects), being overweight, and eating a high-GI processed carbohydrate diet and "bad" fat are the greatest risks for the chronic diseases that plague our lives as we live longer.

THE BODY HAS AN AMAZING CAPACITY TO HEAL ITSELF.

It seems that these are also some of the greatest risk factors for dementia. We know that our genes respond to these factors and produce protective or destructive proteins that alter our destiny. So eating well, exercising, and not smoking will reduce the risk of disease.

New research has also unveiled the role of free radicals as the cause of most chronic diseases, including cancer, arthritis, and dementia. More importantly we are now aware of the importance of antioxidants in the growth of healthy cells, the repair of damaged cells, and the prevention of damage. With this comes the realization that when supplied with optimal nutrition and protected from environmental toxins, the body has an amazing capacity to heal itself. The key to this is a reduction in oxidative stress, a strong immune system, and protection of the cell, particularly the regenerative template, our DNA.

However lucky we might be or how well we may have looked after our health, those who encounter dementia will not see it this way. More and more of us will have to deal with the disease in our closest relatives and friends, our partners, and perhaps ourselves.

> **TO FEEL AND RESPOND TO EMOTION IS INTACT.**

The Lucky Generation has a taste for this life and a sense of entitlement and a distaste for thinking about death. However, the reality of dementia will mean that we will know a new kind of mourning—a mourning for those who have not yet passed on. Loved ones we cannot reach, who cannot know or recognize us, and for whom the present is their only reality as the past no longer exists. It might seem as if their soul has already left them and we are left with only a physical reminder of those we loved and cherished.

And what of the pain, the despair and anguish, of those who suffer the disease? Those who cannot fathom the loss, who cannot summon up the words to express their loneliness as they try to understand who it is they are relating to—apparently their wife or son, they are told? However, tomorrow they will all be strangers again.

But the one thing often left intact is their emotional world. They can feel, and they can laugh and cry. Mostly they suffer in silence as no one can understand their pain. Adults speak of them as if they don't exist, children make jokes and poke fun at them, or else nurses and caregivers just ignore them once they are left in a nursing home to be rendered invisible.

DEMENTIA WILL MEAN A NEW KIND OF MOURNING.

So we have the slow realization that this fate may await us and those we love. To talk about it may seem to hasten a sense of hopeless descent into despair and then grim death. And for this generation, there is a tendency to deny what is happening and a reluctance to talk about it. The message we hear is doom and gloom: our genes will determine our fate, there is no cure, it is inevitable as we grow older. Secretly we know our thinking is not like it used to be; we suspect we become annoyed out of frustration when things are always getting lost or "stolen," but we have our doubts.

Often it is the person's relatives who are the first to talk about the troubling signs. The problems become more evident specially around holiday times when we spend more time together,—or after a partner has died, who covertly made life manageable for their partner and hid the reality from us. Living with this new reality and a seemingly changed person causes fear, confusion, concern, and we need to find out what is happening and what we can do to help—or else just ignore it.

WHO WILL DO THE CARING?

How do we communicate this when feelings are running high and no one wants to accept the reality? Who is going to admit they left the gas on or forgot to turn off a heater, that they have trouble finding the right word or become confused and anxious at family gatherings when everyone is talking at once? These events create doubt, and minds turn to the question of who is going to take responsibility. Who will do the caring when they or we are all too busy with our careers, children, and other interests? It can then seem as if no one cares.

So, how do we talk about dementia when it seems there is no cure? When admitting the problem may signal the loss of independence and ending up in a nursing home—in the trash can waiting to die? Advances in our understanding of the role of the environment and nutrition in the prevention of dementia may provide some hope to those who are showing signs of dementia or who have been diagnosed. I will talk about this later in Chapter 9, as prevention is something that should start as early as possible with the realization that we do have some control.

Chapter 4

Are These Signs of Dementia, or Are We Just Slowing Up a Bit?

Many of us worry that we are getting dementia when we forget things, become a bit grumpy when our routine is changed, or make poor decisions at times. However, this is normal in our later years, or it may mean that we are under stress, suffering some loss, or becoming depressed. When this becomes consistent and noticeable to others, we may have what is called mild cognitive impairment.

> WE HAVE BEEN PROGRAMMED TO FORGET THINGS.

There can be many causes of this, including depression, medication, stress, recent major surgery or a general anesthetic, and many others. In about 10 percent of cases, it can be the precursor of dementia.

When these signs occur, it could be the early stages of dementia. Now might be the time to act, to talk about it and make decisions to change the course of events and take some control of them.

The fact is we have been programmed to forget things or at least not to be consciously aware of much we experience even a short time before. Forgetting makes sense, as, if we recalled everything we did, our minds would become cluttered with useless stuff, and the things we need to know would get crowded out. For example, last month most of us have experienced many pleasurable things: a smile from someone, a nice meal, a chuckle at a cartoon we saw in the paper, the feel of the sun on our face, being intrigued by an interesting program on TV, hearing a good news story on the six o'clock news.

WE NEED TO TOP UP OUR FEEL-GOOD BANK.

Typically, everyday living involves feelings that are positive if we care to notice, though few of us recall the detail: who smiled at you and why, what joke was that, what days were sunny and what days were gloomy, what did you actually eat that tasted so nice, what was that program among many that you liked, and what was that story you heard on the news?

Unless, of course, it was something really special or something we have experienced a few times recently. Otherwise, it comes in and goes out. And tomorrow we will sit down to have another great meal or laugh at a new, or old, joke or watch our favorite TV show. We seem insatiable, as each day we need to get our share of good feelings as if we had never experienced these things before.

So, what use is this, and why do we continually need to experience new things? Surely sunshine today is as good as many other days, this meal no better than many others, that gift is one of many we have received every year of our lives. It seems we need to top up our feel-good bank even when we can't remember what we did a few days earlier.

IT DOESN'T MATTER IF WE FEEL HAPPY AND LOVED.

I believe it is because we have a separate memory system that stores up the good and bad emotions we experience. If we have, or choose to notice, lots of good feelings, we tend to be positive and optimistic, and we tend to expect life to be good. All the negative things don't seem to matter too much. However, if we only experience or choose to focus on negative emotions, we tend to be gloomy and pessimistic, and we expect the worst.

Even as our ability to remember things deteriorates as we age, our emotional memory is still working hard. So it doesn't matter if we can't actually recall the nice things—like a visit from our grandchildren and a birthday cake, a kind word of encouragement, a compliment, an outing with our family—because for a time we feel happy and loved, and it tends to sustain us.

Remember, even when our minds are in tip-top shape, we can't remember what presents we got last year or going on some outing or seeing a movie, but we still do it and we want more. If we have none of these things, but only have experiences that leave us feeling hurt or lonely or unwanted, then we become depressed and sad, even if we can't remember who did what to us or why we felt cold or alone but just that we did, and it grinds us down.

> BY OUR SIXTIES, TIME BETWEEN DOING AND FORGETTING IS SHORTER.

This is even worse when our lives are controlled by others and we cannot do things without support or permission. We cannot just do something just for the fun of it, to feel good for a moment, because we can't. As we become older, our lives become constricted by lack of mobility, lack of resources, or just plain fear and uncertainty about being able to do things on our own.

So what are the signs of dementia. How can we tell the difference between just getting old and the early signs that something more serious is happening. In the next Chapter I explore these issues in some detail.

Chapter 5

What Can We Expect?

By the time we get into our sixties, it's pretty typical that we forget names and appointments, but remember them later; we misplace things like our glasses or keys, but they turn up. The only difference from when we were younger is that the time between doing and forgetting becomes shorter and the amount we can keep in mind at one time is reduced— and it then becomes annoying.

> PEOPLE WITH DEMENTIA MAY FORGET HOW TO GET HOME.

However, the loss associated with dementia is much more profound. One of the most common signs of dementia, especially related to Alzheimer's disease, is memory loss— especially forgetting information we only recently learned and that we need to act on (short-term retrograde memory). Or forgetting to do something in the near future, such as turning off the sprinklers or that we put the kettle on to make a cup of tea (prospective memory).

Although the nature of problems will vary between individuals and even within one individual, memory loss will tend to be a feature of most types of dementia, and it will get worse over time. Depending on the type and progression of the disease, it may be worse for some kinds of material rather than others, for example, verbal and nonverbal information. Other signs may include forgetting important dates or events, asking for the same information over and over, relying on memory aids (e.g., reminder notes or electronic devices) or family members for things people used to be able to handle on their own. It is embarrassing if we wrongly accuse others of stealing something only for it to be found later.

STRESS CAN MAKE PROBLEMS SEEM WORSE

Problems with completing tasks and functioning may not just be about a failure to recall what to do, but can often be attributable to an inability to self-monitor for errors or an inability to develop strategies to perform a previously learned task.

As we get older, most of us lose track of what day of the week it is, particularly when we don't have a set routine, like going to work each day. From time to time, we become tired of obligations such as work and family commitments and need time out when these things overwhelm us to recover our proper functioning. We tend to do this when we have lazy long weekends or when we are on holidays, for example. When we are under pressure or just tired, we may also become aware that we are making poor decisions now and then. Problems can become more apparent if we are under a lot of stress. This is normal.

However, for people with dementia, it is quite a different experience. They can lose track of time, dates, and what season it is, and they can make poor decisions about their spending, like buying unwanted objects or giving money to strangers.

LONELINESS CAN BE A PROBLEM.

They may lose track of once-valued friends and may stop doing things with them that they once enjoyed. Sometimes they may forget where they are or how they got there or how to get home. Inadequate information processing, fatigue, and not being able to focus attention or poor concentration can also affect their memory and behavior.

As we age our hearing deteriorates, we become physically weaker and seeing clearly becomes a nuisance especially when we can never find our glasses!. However, the early stages of dementia may include problems that are not related to physical ailments. These include problems with reading or finding the right word or using the wrong word when we are speaking, judging distance and feeling unsteady on our feet, bumping into objects, particularly on one side of our bodies, or perceiving changes in tone or color. We may start to neglect our hygiene and grooming, not bothering to shave or missing areas or not worrying about doing our hair. We may not notice or not care anymore about stains on our clothes or grime on plates or cutlery. These can often be a source of embarrassment or unease when relatives or friends visit.

DEPRESSION AND ANXIETY CAN CAUSE MEMORY LOSS.

As we age it is inevitable that our friends begin to leave us, and sometimes we lose a partner upon whom we may have come to rely. We are also aware of our diminished capacity to be productive, and sometimes we feel that those around us treat us with disrespect, including health professionals who sometimes speak as if we are not there.

Sometimes changes in mood can be related to medications we are taking, becoming depressed by the change in our functioning and independence, or because of grief when we lose those close to us. Loneliness can be a significant problem when our partner was the primary companion and upon whom we relied. This tends to impact more on women who are suffering from early dementia, as they often depended on their husband. This reliance often meant that relatives have been kept unaware of their declining mental capacity and are, therefore, less able to cope with the disease after he has died. However if we become confused, suspicious, depressed, fearful, or anxious and easily upset at home, at work, with friends, or in other places for little apparent reason, then it may be that these are early signs of dementia.

<hr>

AS WE AGE WE WILL LOSE OUR PARTNER.

<hr>

We know that depression can cause memory loss, inattentiveness, indecisiveness, disorientation, and slower responses, among other things. These signs are commonly referred to as pseudo-dementia. There is a range of treatments to help with the common psychological problems, but you need to know they are not early symptoms of dementia, as apathy, considered a symptom of dementia, looks very much like depression.

One important difference is that older people with depression tend to lose interest in or lose the ability to enjoy normal activities. Whereas the person with dementia, particularly in the early stages, can derive pleasure from such things as seeing grandchildren and participating in some celebration.

Often your memory problems can be just a part of the normal aging process. We also tend to think and react more slowly as we age. However, we sometimes do our best work when we use all the experience we have gained over our lives, as long-term memory is rarely affected by aging and may, in fact, improve. Sometimes we find it hard to learn new things or to plan as well as we used to, but we can still enjoy many aspects of our lives despite the declining years. Worrying needlessly only takes from our lives and may turn into depression and anxiety.

THE TIME COMES WHEN SUPPORT WILL BE NECESSARY.

As we age there is a good chance, especially if we are female, that we will lose our partner. A sense of loss is at the center of dealing with a loved one with dementia, but also for people with the disease who become aware of failing capacity to cope and manage their lives. Therefore, feelings of grief can be a significant issue as we find it difficult to deal with the reality of dementia and what it means. Sometimes a psychologist or psychotherapist can help you through this difficult time of loss and adjustment.

Common to different forms of dementia, significant problems may include language and communication. Therefore, effective interventions to improve functioning can be compromised when communication breaks down. Issues of concern include word-finding problems, difficulty focusing on the topic, poor turn-taking, talkativeness, difficulties sustaining conversation because of difficulties forming ideas, difficulties following discussions where there is noise or when many people are talking at once, lack of tact and inappropriate comments, trouble understanding abstract ideas, and repetition of observations. Other problems include an inability to pick up on nonverbal cues, difficulties maintaining a sense of context, and problems with logical argument. Maintaining interest and concentration can appear as if language is impaired if people cannot follow a conversation or deal with distractions. Communication can be difficult due to unclear speech, speech rate, and volume.

TALKING ABOUT DEMENTIA IS IMPORTANT.

Some forms of dementia are marked by poor interpersonal skills and distressing behaviors, including outbursts of anger or inappropriate laughter, inappropriate touching, or sexually explicit conduct. Antisocial acts such as impulsivity, self-centeredness, attention-seeking, and manipulative behavior can be very distressing for caregivers as they often represent changes in responses that are quite different from before individuals had dementia, especially when the behaviors are not recognized as being a symptom of dementia. Similarly apathy and a lack of motivation can be confusing and lead to conflict.

The next chapter of this book focuses on the benefits of talking about dementia with our loved ones at an early stage. Importantly it describes how we can achieve that sensitively and effectively to achieve the best possible quality of life in the future.

Chapter 6

Talking about Dementia

There are some excellent reasons to talk about dementia. Finding out as early as possible if a person has dementia can have significant benefits. The most important benefit is that things that can be done to slow its progress and to enhance continued quality of life. For example, exercise and socialization have been found to increase functioning and delay onset; some medications can cause dementia-like symptoms or make them worse; high blood pressure and cholesterol can increase the risk of dementia; diet and nutrition can be essential, as well as remaining active or even having the occasional alcoholic drink.

DOCTORS MAY NOT WANT TO TALK ABOUT DEMENTIA.

Despite the current lack of effective treatment, recognition of early-stage dementia may offer substantial benefits. These include avoidance of inappropriate treatment related to misdiagnosis and time for you and your family to address issues of support services, accommodation, and financial, legal, and medical-care planning.

The symptoms associated with dementia need to be thoroughly investigated and treated, as there are many preventable causes of dementia or things that share some of the symptoms and signs. They include: an abnormal growth of tissue, either benign or sometimes malignant like the various tumors or cancers; high or low chemical levels in the blood; vitamin deficiencies; thyroid disease; hormone level changes; kidney or liver disease; head injury; alcohol and toxic chemicals (heavy metals and pesticides); a range of brain diseases like meningitis; autoimmune disease like lupus; both prescribed drugs (anticholinergics, antidepressants) and alcohol and illicit drug abuse; mental illness (depression and anxiety); and many others.

PERSONAL ISSUES AND EMOTIONS CAN BE OUT-OF-BOUNDS.

The most important preventive strategy is to facilitate repair and generation of healthy cells. To prevent damage, cells need a generous supply of nutrients and an ability to defend against oxidative stress that causes damage to cells.

In discussions of dementia, knowing these things and being able to communicate that while we still can can make a big difference to how we are treated. Getting treatment is important. We may even have to educate our doctors because many don't know this, and many are reluctant to talk about it because they feel inadequate not being able to help and because they know how much distress a diagnosis can cause. Moreover, the course of the disease is unpredictable, so there is a reluctance to answer some questions directly. Symptoms can be influenced by other health problems, personality, family support, and coping ay, as well as intellectual attainments before onset of symptoms. As a result the decline can be slow and gradual or rapid, leading to death in only a few years after onset. Many doctors, due to the emphasis on treatment rather than prevention, ignore the growing evidence that factors such as exercise, diet, and nutritional supplements can play a vital role in the prevention of many chronic diseases.

EMPATHY CAN BE CONVEYED BY GENUINE INTEREST.

The most recognized chronic disease is type 2 diabetes, which is the result of insulin resistance and is directly related to lifestyle choices. It is highly likely that these same factors may play a role in dementia. As well as talking in chapter 11 about what we as professionals can provide, in this chapter I spend some time talking about the importance of good communication with the person with dementia as the first step in providing adequate and respectful treatment. Caregivers may benefit from reading this section and also in determining if the professional you go to is on the job.

An issue of fundamental importance in talking about dementia is to assume competence and to focus on the abilities of the individual who develops dementia. In doing this we are taking care of the feelings of the one we care about. To focus on symptoms or disability and to take over the person's life is demeaning and destructive of their sense of self-worth. Ultimately it is most important to have a realistic view of what is to come and to be prepared.

SHE DEVOTED HERSELF TO CARING FOR HER MOTHER

I treated a young woman who had been diagnosed with depression related to grieving for the loss of her mother. However, her mother had passed away some three years before, and her life was almost entirely dysfunctional. She found it hard to leave the house, she was filled with a deep sense of dread that something would happen to her or her loved ones, and she spent most of her time lost in meaningless worry, staring at a TV that was not turned on. Mostly she felt it was pointless to do anything, and she derived no pleasure from any activity and often thought of her death.

She had grown up in Zimbabwe. It was a time of great social upheaval, with a constant threat of violence, especially for a young girl. While she felt little apprehension growing up in this environment, her mother watched her and carefully supervised her life to protect her from harm. Since then her family came to Australia to take up farming here. Despite the greater safety here it emerged as we talked together that she had stayed very close to her mother and become very reliant on her for her sense of well-being. When she was at boarding school, her mother was diagnosed with dementia even though she was only fifty-five.

> ### SHE HAD NOT TALKED ABOUT HER MOTHER DYING.

When things became very difficult she then gave up her university study even though she was in her final year to help her father care for her mother. For some years she devoted herself to caring for her mother. In desperation they turned to alternative therapies she felt would help her mother recover, and for a period the symptoms seemed to abate.

She then met someone special and went away with him for a few months. While she was away overseas, her mother died. She said she was completely devastated and blamed herself. From that day, she could not live normally. She lost interest in doing anything, she struggled to go to work each day, she spent and lot of time crying and not getting out of bed. Her relationship became strained. She also pondered on her own death and saw it as a solution to her mental suffering. It became apparent that her father and she had not talked about the possibility of her mother dying. She could now see that everyone except her understood that and was prepared. Because of her denial, she could not deal with her mother's death. By talking about the reality of dementia, of her attachment to her mother, and her lack of the ability to talk openly about the disease, she started to recover.

UNDERSTANDING THE PERSON'S EXPERIENCE IS EMPATHY.

There are a few fundamental principles for good communication. This can be difficult dealing with people who are often defensive about what is happening to them. They are often in a state of denial and worry about your motives for wanting to know something. In some families, discussion of these personal issues is out-of-bounds. Some families avoid talking about or experiencing emotions together. But now is the time to enter new territory and to find a way to talk about some crucial stuff that can't wait.

The first principle is empathy. To empathize means not assuming that you know how the other person is feeling or experiencing the dementia. Instead, it is an attempt to step outside your concerns and to be with them in their apprehension, fear, and sense of loss and despair. Empathy can be conveyed by our genuine interest in what they have to say. To do this we maintain attention, we are open in the way we present ourselves, and we signal that we have heard by affirmation, by repeating what we believe they have said, by asking questions better to understand the particular meaning attached to words and nonverbal signs. We signal our positive regard for the person by making them aware that we see their good qualities, not just the bad things that are happening. We should refrain from giving unasked-for advice and discounting their needs and preferences.

THE 'DIAGNOSIS' OF DEMENTIA CAN BE PREMATURE.

Often the person with dementia does not understand or can be terribly afraid about what is happening to them. They may be worried about others' reactions and what others may have in store for them, or about being an unwanted burden. As a consequence they may make up stories or act in a way that helps them make sense of things unknown.

Story-making like this is not lying or being devious; it is often the best they can do to make sense of something that is frightening. To make sense of something means that it can seem less fearful. Attempting to understand the reason for a person thinking or doing something that may appear nonsensical to you is a measure of the level of empathy you can have. By being dismissive or imposing our "rational" thinking, we demonstrate contempt for the person we want to help, even if we never meant that to be the case.

INCREASED TRUST HELPS US ASK DIFFICULT QUESTIONS.

I recently saw a family in crisis. The two elder children believed their mother was suffering from dementia and feared for her safety, especially since she was living alone in the large family home since their father had died. They had sold the house and moved her from Melbourne to Sydney to stay in a one-bedroom flat that was close to their homes. Despite visiting her each week and organizing for some day care, it seemed that her functioning had deteriorated. She seemed more forgetful, indecisive, and fuzzy-headed.

I first saw her with her younger daughter, who had come from the country to Sydney to visit her mother. She was convinced that her mother did not have dementia but was lonely and grieving, not just at the loss of her husband of forty-five years, but of all her friends and the familiarity of the suburb she had lived in most of her life. When I saw her, I, too, agreed with both the daughter and mother that she did not appear to have significant cognitive problems.

She was coherent, and she spoke clearly and movingly about the recent loss of her husband and the disruptive nature of her move. She understood her elder children meant well but could not help but feel the wrong choice had been made, despite being so far from her family. When we all got together at a later session to try to come to some better arrangement, I witnessed a marked change in her functioning and behavior.

In the presence of her older children, she seemed to lose confidence; she spoke with hesitancy and appeared to get lost.

> CONFRONTATION MAKES CLEAR WHAT IS NOT BEING TALKED ABOUT.

She began to dither and, her eyes downcast, she lapsed into silence and let them talk over her and about her. With the help and reassurance of the younger daughter, it became possible for her to start to talk about her sadness and loneliness. She also began to talk about how ungrateful she felt, but also of her fears that she might be abandoned by her children if they felt she was not able to adapt. She had heard them talking about her "dementia" and their fears for her. But instead of being reassured, this made her more fearful. The dreadful thought that she would lose her mind and end up totally alone and at the mercy of strangers in a "home" made her withdraw further and ironically to adopt the role.

I referred her to a psychologist colleague who spent some time helping her deal with the multiple losses in her life since her husband's passing and her move to Sydney. She also became involved as a volunteer in a local historical society and started to make some new friends. It seems that the "diagnosis" of dementia her family had provided was a bit premature. Loneliness, grief, and fear were her problems, and these had been discounted by those who too readily applied a label that so often is wrong.

DIFFICULT QUESTIONS NEED TO BE ASKED

As can be seen from the example above, there are excellent practical reasons for developing rapport or empathy: we develop trust. Trust is the second principle of effective communication. Without some measure of trust, we cannot feel comfortable about being vulnerable, as it can be used to hurt us. Increased confidence in each other tends to reduce levels of anxiety and enable us to ask the difficult questions that need to be asked. Having the courage to do so may allow people with dementia to open up to the point where they may be able to think more clearly about the reasons for their behavior and to start to talk about their feelings.

More than this, it allows us the opportunity to confront the person with the reality of what is happening and the need to do something. Confrontation is the third fundamental principle. Confrontation does not mean that what we say is negative, hurtful, or derogatory, but it can make clear what seems apparent but is not being talked about. Now this can be risky, as we may be wrong about the point we want to make or what we might want to achieve.

ADVICE GIVING IS NOT THE BEST WAY TO BUILD RAPPORT.

However, if we have developed a good level of trust and it is understood that we have acted in good faith, then misunderstanding may not be a bad thing, and in fact, it may add to what we know or do not know. The very act of speaking frankly and showing the courage to take a risk can reveal our vulnerability.

The level of intimacy can be deepened if the person you care about has answered without being defensive and feels safe in talking openly and being vulnerable, just as you are. When effective communication occurs, the nature of the relationship has deepened, and a greater level of mutual respect has occurred.

Advice giving is not the best way to build rapport. Often it signals that we don't have the time or patience to stop and listen. It signals we don't want to understand what is happening from the other's point of view and that we discount his or her attempts to deal with the problem and that we know better. In the end it is often insulting and demeaning, suggesting that the other does not have the wits to work out what to do for his or her own welfare. It assumes far too much knowledge.

AN ADVANCED-CARE DIRECTIVE MAY BE DESIRABLE

On the other hand, having built a trusting relationship, it may be timely to look at options and to involve your loved one in a meaningful way in a discussion of what choices he or she has. Not to have this talk may result in grave consequences if the issues are left unresolved.

At this time it is possible to talk about failing health, loss of mental faculties, the need to depend on others for survival, the loss of dignity and independence, and death. Preparation for the inevitable decline and then passing from this world awaits us all, but as it draws near, it assumes a level of gravity that is easily ignored when we are young and healthy.

Many issues need to be addressed, like writing an advanced-care directive, drawing up a will and choosing an executor, making arrangements for income protection and the possible sale of assets, and deciding where to live so that adequate care is available.

Perhaps appointing an enduring guardian and someone to assume responsibility for financial and other legal responsibilities can all be planned for in an orderly way. All this allows full participation by the person with dementia if done early enough with the assurance that his or her desires are honored and his or her rights protected.

> INVOLVE YOUR LOVED ONE IN DISCUSSING CHOICES.

Also a realistic appraisal of the stage of dementia, what other health issues are present, the need for and appropriateness of treatment, and the role of health professionals can be considered and acted upon in a timely fashion.

In chapter 8 I want to address the complexity of caring for someone with dementia and what this means and then talk more about the treatment options that are possible in chapter 12. And I talk about legal issues in some detail in chapter 14. However, in the next chapter, I want to address the issues of grief and loss.

Chapter 7

Grief and Dementia

It's said that time will heal. However, as with grief following the death of a loved one, it is not time that leads to a resolution of the pain, but the process that occurs during this period.

The process of resolving grief is to confront the feelings and thoughts that are continually at play, rather than to ignore them or try to push them away. Keeping these sensations at bay by using drugs, distractions, or willpower only delays the need to deal with these painful feelings and thoughts at some later time.

> CARING CAN ALLOW A NEW LEVEL OF INTIMACY.

It is now well-established that grief responses follow loss or separation. Death is the most obvious loss, and grief is a natural consequence of bonds of affection being lost. Separation for whatever reason can also precipitate the same feelings of grief and bereavement, not just between parents and children, but between sexual partners and even between siblings. The heart of affectionate bonding or attachment is care-giving and care receiving. When the loss involves dementia, it is a separation that most often fundamentally changes the caregiving/care-receiving process. Most often it is the parent who has provided care and nurturance over a lifetime. Not only is this process curtailed, but also it often involves reversal of roles, with the caretaker now being called upon to provide the care. A profound sense of alienation and anxiety at the loss of a relationship that nurtured a sense of safety and certainty manifests as grief.

WE CANNOT EXPECT AN INTELLIGENT CONVERSATION

Moreover, in the case of someone with dementia, the passing of time tends to increase the sense of loss, alienation, and sadness. The need to find a sense of acceptance and peace during this time is even more important. That process involves learning to relate to your loved one with dementia in a different way. Without diminishing the character and status of the person with dementia or trivializing the situation, I believe that the process of relating to a two-year-old has significant similarities to the way we might relate when memory and mind are affected by dementia.

We cannot expect to hold a rational or intelligent conversation with a two-year-old. Therefore, we cannot expect the same level of support or reliance that we became used to over many years from our adult relative or loved one. Things have changed. However, we can derive enormous pleasure by reassessing our needs and adapting for ourselves a new type of communication that involves few words, but comprises love and affection, patience, high emotional content, touching, cuddling, and play. The benefit for the person with dementia is even more important in terms of emotional well-being and quality of life.

> CARING FOR HIS FATHER WAS A TURNING POINT IN HIS LIFE.

The need to do this for the person with dementia is even more necessary. Moving from grieving to resolution may well involve a process that can bring a sense of peace to your lives despite the loss of all that the relationship once represented. In other words, not only is there a need to confront the loss, but also to refashion the relationship to bring this about.

A patient I saw some years ago talked about a new level of intimacy and richness gained by taking on the role of caring for his father in the last year of the father's life. After work he would come to his family home and feed and bathe his father and put him into bed. Then he would sit with his mother and talk about the father and husband and all he had given them. He had known his father as a generous, accomplished, and outgoing, larger-than-life character from whom he had learned much and on whom he had depended for much of his life for mentoring and direction.

He spoke with tears in his eyes of the satisfaction he gained by gently washing and dressing the man for whom he had a deep affection. They couldn't speak, but the communication was more meaningful than he had ever experienced. It was also a turning point in his life. In recent times, with success and money and wealthy friends, he had begun using cocaine.

> ### RESTRUCTURING HIS LIFE MEANT EMBRACING HIS FATHER'S ILLNESS.

He had come to me to help stop what he saw as destructive and contrary to the values his father had tried to instill. The motivation to use drugs was not just indulgence. He had unknowingly done so to help him deal with the disturbing feelings that threatened to overcome him since his father started to descend into the world of dementia.

His nurturing of his father in these months enabled him to understand the reason he started using drugs and allowed him to reject that as an option. He was also due to become a father himself and hoped his father would be alive to see his new grandson. That was not possible as his father died three weeks before the baby was born; however, his commitment to his role as a father had taken a new direction since he started caring for his father. He had managed to restructure his life as a result of the closeness he had experienced with his father. His capacity to confront and deal with his grief when his father did die was no doubt made more meaningful by their time together. The pain of his loss was no less—in fact, it was probably more acute—but it would pass, and he would be left with fond memories of their days together.

> ## HE COULD NOT DEAL WITH THE CHANGE IN HIS FATHER

On the other hand, his elder brother had become angry and embittered by his father's "abandonment." He could not bring himself to be with him as he had changed so much from the man he had known for some forty years. The man he no longer recognized filled him with a sense of revulsion. He could not confront and deal with the change in his father or the change he needed to make to properly resolve his grief. His father's eventual passing only compounded his anger and sense of betrayal.

The process of restructuring my patient's life was based on his capacity to embrace his father and his illness and to adopt an entirely different view of their relationship and mode of that interaction. It was a process his brother could not accept. To him his father was no longer the nurturing mentor and guide, but the helpless child. He was no longer the indulgent son who relied on his father, but he had found a new role and purpose as caregiver.

> HIS FATHER WAS NO LONGER A MENTOR AND GUIDE.

As this story illustrates, it is not purely a matter of engagement in other activities that may lessen the pain. More so, it is an involvement in some meaningful activity that embraces the reality of dementia and eventual passing. It is true that few events are powerful enough to displace the pain and the ever constant worries. More than that, for the person who is grieving a loss, few activities appear to be attractive or worthwhile even starting.

What can be achieved with the resolution of grief goes to the heart of this story. It may seem obvious that the aim is to get rid of the emotional pain and tormenting thoughts: to find relief from uncomfortable and unwanted feelings. In other words, to return to what we knew and felt comfortable with before the loss. Of course, this is not possible, for with some events, change precludes going back.

I was recently seeing a forty-five-year-old married woman who had relapsed to alcohol binging. She had seen me some years before for the same problem. At that time the alcoholism largely came about due to the slow development of a problem of using alcohol to deal with many of the self-imposed pressures in her life. Whatever the reason for starting, an addiction results from the continued heavy use of alcohol or a drug or behavior such as gambling or Internet porn.

THE THINKING BRAIN IS HIJACKED BY DRUGS

This process involves slow structural changes in the brain, as the activity hijacks the unconscious survival pathways in the brain. The midbrain commands control, motivation, and reward pathways, and it regulates such activities as hunger, thirst, sex, security, and other essential survival activities for the person and species.

When alcohol use or other rewarding activities are repeated often enough, these activities become salient or preferred behavior. Repeated action quickly and reliably rewards and reinforces these pathways lying deep within our subconscious. When that happens our capacity to weigh the consequences of the behavior is distorted or absent, and addictive behavior is continued even though we are aware of the sometimes severe negative consequences. The thinking part of our brain, which is not directly connected to the environment, is cut off, and we are driven by these hijacked "survival" mechanisms. In other words, we lose control of the behavior despite it being self-destructive of the organism.

The lady again sought my help as she had recently realized that her mother was developing dementia and she had started to drink again. This time her marriage was on the line. No matter what the reason, her husband was not going to tolerate any more of her drunken behavior.

> HER WORLD WAS TURNED UPSIDE DOWN WITH MULTIPLE LOSSES.

She was deeply distressed for many reasons, but it was mainly the realization that her mother, who she had depended on the most and who was her trusted confidante was no longer able to take that role. As her mother became more disconnected from the world, so her sense of isolation and aloneness became more pronounced, and she sought comfort in drinking. It is well-documented that the more intense a relationship, the more profound the grief. In this case her father had died when she was five, and as an only child, she and her mother had developed a very close bond upon which she came to rely. She described it as more like having an older sister she could confide in.

In recent times she had relied on her mother more than ever as her relationship with her husband became more strained. Over the preceding ten years, her mother was always there if her children needed caring for, she needed an extra hand for a dinner party, or most importantly, if she needed to share her most intimate feelings.

> ## SHE FEARED FOR HER MOTHER'S SAFETY.

Not only was her mother now needing her help, but her children were now completing high school. She had always waited on them, hand and foot, but now they did not need her as they asserted their independence...unless it was to get a lift somewhere or needing some money for some activity that excluded her!

Her world was being turned upside down with multiple losses of relationships as her identity as defined by these relationships. Moreover, her role and sense of purpose were also threatened with the prospect that her relationship with her husband was in jeopardy.

Moreover, her mother's responses were confusing for her. Some days the mother seemed to be fine as her long-term memory was mostly intact. Other days she felt devastated as she realized that her mother was not able to recall a conversation from a day or so before, or her perceptions were becoming distorted, her behavior erratic, and most alarmingly, she realized that her mother's safety was being compromised. While the mother was still driving, she noticed that sometimes her mother would take hours to find her way home from shopping at the local supermarket.

HER MOTHER WAS NOW RELIANT ON HER.

The immediate goal of therapy was to stop the drinking, and this was primarily accomplished by her taking naltrexone tablets daily, as this medication dramatically reduces craving for alcohol. With the drinking under control, we looked at the conditioned triggers to drink and removed them as much as possible and then gradually exposed her to them: for example, taking a different route home from shopping that avoided the bottle shop. The next task (worked on concurrently) was to help her understand the nature of her highly dependent relationship with her mother and to develop a new basis for that relationship that meant she was the caregiver and that her mother was now reliant on her.

She also needed to find new roles that gave her life meaning, and she resumed part-time work in her old job. While the pay was not great, it was very satisfying reestablishing her friendships at work. She also volunteered to do some work for Alzheimer's Australia so she could learn more about caring for someone with dementia and better equip herself when her mother would need much more of her time. At the same time, we worked on her feelings of loss and grief. She mourned the passing of one phase of her life and the need to transition to a new reality that in many ways would be just as fulfilling, although very different.

SOMETIMES THE LOSS APPEARS TOO DIFFICULT TO BEAR.

The final task was to work on deepening the intimacy with her husband and reestablishing the trust that had been damaged over many years of alcohol abuse. The counseling work was very much about her learning to share her feelings with him, a role her mother had taken on for too long. He not only felt alienated by her drinking, but by being left out of her most private life that he thought he should have been a part of.

However, as it emerged in this case, we realized that what looked like resolution can be displacement and preoccupation, often accompanied by an ongoing sense of disquiet and anxiety. In therapy these issues were worked over many times until we felt confident that a new way of being with her mother and husband were internalized. If this doesn't happen, the sense of loss can be suppressed and manifest in destructive ways. In this case it manifested as alcohol dependence; even worse, it can manifest as illness and death for the grieving person who finds it impossible to resolve the pain or to relinquish the dependence on the demented person. They struggle to find new meanings and attachments in their lives, particularly if other relationships have been diminished by the preoccupation with the other.

> ## RESOLUTION OF GRIEF IS A PROCESS OF GROWTH.

My patient will continue to struggle with her sense of loss and her need to find others to share her sense of loss, as well as to understand herself and to maintain her sense of identity and worth. While this evolves she will need support not to relapse to alcohol use, which threatened to destroy her life.

Sometimes the loss appears to be too difficult to bear or to overcome. Loss can also lead to self-blame, isolation, and an inability to detach from the need for the type of relationship that existed, leading to disinterest in normal activities.

When a close relationship is lost, the capacity to resolve the grief may be derailed by constant rumination of the loss and desperate efforts to relieve the pain, as we saw in the story above. The emotional experience can be akin to the way we deal with trauma, which involves a loss of meaning and a sense of safety that was reflected in the experience of the young woman from Zimbabwe. Unless we can integrate the new reality into a new worldview and a new way of being in the world, it will seem disconnected from reality and be a constant source of anxiety. Staying stuck with one way of viewing the event is dysfunctional and unlikely to lead to progress and resolution.

DEMENTIA CAN LEAD TO ISOLATION FOR THE CAREGIVER.

In the case of a loved one with dementia, the daily round of caring and worry does not lessen, and the constant challenges and instances of distress always remind us of the emotional pain of loss and rejection.

To make this burden and suffering relevant or meaningful seems almost impossible, as there is no relief. As a means of dealing with other pressing demands and as a distraction, as well as recovering lost energy and providing other meaningful outlets, respite care can provide temporary relief. However, psychological help may be needed to negotiate this difficult time and find new ways of reestablishing a sense of identity and a sense of purpose and safety.

Ultimately the resolution of grief depends on our ability for growth as a person. More pragmatically it is a capacity to integrate what can be a profoundly disturbing shift in reality. Change leaves us disoriented and afraid and greatly at odds with the new reality we have generated in our being through our living experience. With the change comes uncertainty and an inability to confidently predict what fate awaits us.

DEMENTIA REMINDS US OF OUR MORTALITY AND FRAILTY.

Dementia for the caregiver can lead to isolation and loss of friendships, to loneliness and a change of social status. And with uncertainty comes fear. With a disease like dementia, it conjures up our mortality and frailty in a way that we have learned to put to one side and to pretend won't happen. Resolution is a capacity to look to the time when we are similarly brought to the brink of our life and to be able to view it with some sense of equanimity and grace.

In the next chapter of this book, I want to talk about some practical things that families can do to care for their elderly loved ones.

Chapter 8

What Can Families Do?

Early and accurate detection can make a lot of difference to people's lives. Firstly, the symptoms of concern may not be dementia, just changes that occur with age; it may be psychological problems that make it harder to remember, concentrate, and make decisions; it may that their excessive alcohol consumption over a number of years has affected the brain (and it might be time to stop). In any case it is important to know about this so you and your family can plan ahead and make some important decisions while your loved one can still fully participate.

THEY CAN STILL FEEL AND THEIR FEELINGS MATTER

It is vitally important that as your loved ones grow older and more vulnerable, they are able to make some choices about their future. Most often dementia is associated with depression and anxiety (which make symptoms worse). Losses they may experience can worsen if others make choices for them they may find fearful or hard to deal with. They might not be able to care for themselves completely and they may forget things but they can still feel, and they need you to understand that their feelings are still important even when they find it hard to tell anyone. Planning will give them the sense that they are still in control of what might happen to them, including the chance of being moved to a nursing home away from all that is familiar and important to them.

WHAT IS IMPOSED IS NOT VALUED OR WANTED.

It is also important that when we talk to those we are concerned about, we actually talk to them as if they matter, not just to each other as if they don't exist. By using the skills for honest and effective communication based on the principles I talked about in chapter 6, we may be able to talk frankly about the future and to encourage our loved ones to be involved in the plans that are necessary to implement. They must be allowed to make choices about what they want to talk about and the things that affect them. It is their choice as to who gets any results of assessment, what they are capable and not capable of, and what is done with this knowledge. It is their choice as to what they would like to achieve, what goals to set, and what they might enjoy doing. Otherwise, it is imposed and not valued or wanted.

At the same time, it is important to the person with dementia to have those who care about them share from their perspective how they are coping. This is so the person with dementia gets a broad view of the problems the caregivers may have in daily living. Sometimes it is really important for you as caregivers to talk to the person with dementia about your needs. Some things, like having time for others and for yourself, you may regard as being important so that you can cope.

ASSESSMENT OF PAIN CAN BE DIFFICULT.

Sometimes you are just as confused and distressed about what is happening as they are, but mostly you want to be able to help them to improve their quality of life and functioning and to retain the relationship as long as possible. At the same time, you need to protect yourself and the interests of others who might depend on you.

As well as memory problems and getting lost, as discussed earlier, serious language problems can develop, although different problems can mean different things. For example, can the person with dementia speak to you, is their speech slurred or hard to understand, or do they have trouble finding the right words? Different symptoms can indicate what areas of the brain are damaged and, therefore, the relative impact on being able to communicate successfully.

Over 60 percent of people with dementia are also suffering from depression. Not only can depression contribute to a number of significant problems, but it can make worse the severity of dementia-like symptoms; for those who can't communicate other issues like acute or chronic pain, their inability to communicate can be mistaken for an unwillingness to cooperate or a desire to complain for no apparent reason.

LATE STAGE DEMENTIA REQUIRES CONSTANT CARE.

For people with unrecognized pain, there may be a perception that there is a reluctance to treat, and therefore no relief from the pain can be attributed to the lack of care by health professionals, like not getting the medication people think they need and not being admitted to the hospital for treatment—which also leads to the belief that they are not being heard or their needs taken seriously. A person in pain can be ground down by it and sink further into depression and their levels of energy deplete, creating a downward spiral.

Even for professionals, in people with dementia, mental impairment or communication problems mean that assessment of pain can be difficult and sometimes result in inadequate levels of pain relief. This may be despite the best efforts of caregivers to understand and explain the limits of what they can do and what is effective and appropriate treatment. All this will cause the people with dementia to feel very frustrated and despairing as they feel they are losing control of their lives.

Once dementia has become serious and the person needs constant care, then decline can be quite rapid. Not much can be done to treat dementia by this stage. For example, if they have vascular dementia, then treatment to reduce blood pressure might be suggested. It is unlikely to be helpful as those areas of the brain that have been denied sufficient blood flow will not recover lost function.

DO WHAT BRINGS PLEASURE AS LONG AS POSSIBLE

By the time Alzheimer's disease is diagnosed, serious damage has already occurred in 60 percent of the memory centers of the brain. However, you need to know if any other condition or medication is making symptoms worse, such as infections or anticholinergic drugs. The GP can check this out when you seek professional help.

I think the important thing to remember is your loved ones can still feel and their emotional responses are still likely to be intact. Depression being so common in people with dementia indicates that, I believe. It is important for as long as possible for them to do things that give them pleasure. To do things that they enjoy, like having their favorite food, having a pet, or listening to music they have always liked, even if they just play the same thing over and over again. Sometimes recordings of happy messages from their children or grandchildren or other loved ones who cannot be around them can bring pleasure. Especially talking about things that happened earlier in their lives as their long-term memory is probably a lot less affected than their short-term memory. It's also good if their loved ones can come and be with them. If not then they can play them when you can't be there.

EMOTIONAL RESPONSES ARE OFTEN INTACT.

While this may seem like time wasted if they can't remember you being there, it will bring pleasure. Children and grandchildren need to be reminded of this and encouraged to visit for their sake.

Even if it seems they can't remember doing something, it doesn't matter. If they feel good about something, can smile, and let you know they feel a bit of relief from their pain or sadness, then they will tend to remember this in a different way, and their depression may not be so bad.

At this stage of their lives, it is all about allowing them some enjoyment. It is sad to see them decline and suffer, but I guess you need to be there for them and remember to do what you can to make each day as happy as it can be.

There are government schemes that can pay for assistance for families and their loved ones, including cleaning, shopping, and so on, and also providing some time off from caring if it gets to be too much.

SUPPORT AGENCIES CAN PROVIDE INFORMATION AND SUPPORT

You may need to contact the local community health center and have an assessment team come and assess them for eligibility.

There are private support agencies and organizations like Alzheimer's Australia and Dementia Care Australia that can provide information, support, and treatment programs like Alzheimer's Australia's Living with Memory Loss program. Contact details can be found in the Resources list at the end of this book on page 184.

Families also need to be aware of the safety of their loved one as well as their own safety, as the loved one may forget to turn things like heaters or taps off or lose balance and fall. Again, having some assistance can be important for you to see that they don't suffer more than they have to and for you to get some relief from the worry and the effort you must put in to help your loved one.

Relatives tend to suffer sadness and feelings of loss that resemble grief and confusion when loved ones decline. The emergence of deeply disturbing feelings often relates to no longer having the practical support and companionship of the person with dementia.

FEELINGS RESEMBLING GRIEF CAN BE CONFUSING.

Perhaps more so, the loss of the person they once knew and cherished, who is in many respects no longer here, and of abandonment and withdrawal of love as the individual with dementia appears detached and unconcerned. Feelings resembling grief, such as yearning and preoccupation, anger, blame, guilt, sadness, distress, and anxiety, can be confusing and debilitating and misunderstood by others. Arranging with your GP for you to see a psychologist to talk about what you are going through and how you can care for yourself will help you cope and help your loved one as well. No good you falling into a heap!

In addition to the severe decline in functioning, a usual consequence of dementia, there are a number of conditions that mimic symptoms of dementia. Some things can make symptoms worse or bring about significant problems that are not related to the dementia. Moreover, some are treatable. Apart from the relief of unnecessary suffering this can bring, it is important to determine this, as some conditions left untreated can have serious consequences.

> **THE AIM OF TREATMENT IS TO COMPENSATE FOR LOST CAPACITY.**

If there are indications or signs of other complicating issues, this can allow health professionals to include these in treatment planning to design programs to reduce the impact on the health and well-being of the person with dementia.

While dementia is virtually incurable, progress can be delayed, functioning maintained, and quality of life improved for the person with dementia and their caregivers for some time. However, in later stages of the disease, thoughts of cure, reversal of symptoms, or rehabilitation are inappropriate, and to suggest this is possible is only offering false hope. Interventions should be concerned with an improvement in functioning to the extent that this is possible, and optimizing quality of life for as long as possible.

The aim of treatment and support then becomes a matter of compensating for lost capacity. It is achieved by emphasizing and working with the abilities that are still intact, simplifying, modifying, or avoiding some tasks, changing the environment, and providing appropriate external support services. I talk at length about improving quality of life in the later stages of dementia in Chapter 13.

LIFESTYLE CHANGES CAN PREVENT DEMENTIA

Moreover, with this knowledge you can help them take control of their lives and implement plans for their future at a time when they were able to make clear what it is that they want. When a disease progresses beyond a certain point cure becomes very difficult or impossible. This realization highlights the essential importance of prevention to optimize our health. At a much earlier stage, there is an opportunity to make lifestyle changes that can prevent dementia.

The next chapter of this book will focus on the development of these strategies and how they are to be achieved, with a particular focus on exercise, diet, nutrition, and changing patterns of behavior.

Chapter 9

Prevention of Dementia: What We Can Do Now?

Changes in lifestyle, such as quitting smoking, reducing weight, and lowering high blood pressure can reduce the risk and perhaps delay onset and slow the progress of dementia. We now think keeping an active mind may not only reduce the risk, but may allow people to cope with dementia better and to function at a higher level for longer.

> MODERN LIFE CAUSES ANXIETY AND STRESS.

Along with regular, moderate exercise, nutrition is of vital importance, with research showing that certain substances are crucial to brain function and health. Increased blood flow to the brain provides essential requirements such as oxygen and glucose, which provide the energy for neurons to work, vitamins and minerals to ensure proper firing of neurons, and enzyme function and antioxidants to protect cells and maintain the health of the brain.

Moreover, evidence shows that by adopting lifestyle changes, exercising, eating healthily, and taking good-quality supplements can prevent many chronic diseases, including dementia. This chapter focuses on prevention:

what we can do before the onset of chronic disease and even after we detect early signs.

All of us are subject to the effect of the pollutants in the air we breathe. Some intake of toxins can be significantly reduced, such as avoiding cigarette smoke and car exhaust fumes. However, some pollutants are a product of our way of life, such as air pollution, radioactivity, and petrochemicals in insecticides and plastic manufacture. We are all impacted by radiation directly from the sun or background radiation in the natural and urban environment.

NUTRITION AND EXERCISE DECREASES THE RISK BY 45%.

The pace of modern life means that we are often feeling anxious and stressed. All of these can impact on our bodies, causing oxidative stress and hastening the chances of getting dementia and other diseases such as arthritis and cancer. Antioxidants, fatty acids, vitamins, and minerals have been shown to reverse some of these effects.

The ground rules to ensure a healthy diet and adequate nutrition are to eat a variety of foods from each food category (proteins, carbohydrates, and fats), maintain a healthy weight through a proper balance of exercise and food, choose foods low in saturated fat, and eliminate as far as possible processed carbohydrates (high GI), including sugar, white rice, and bread, as well as moderate the use of salt, drink eight glasses of water per day, drink alcohol in moderation, and include foods high in antioxidant content.

It seems the ancient practitioners of Traditional Chinese Medicine understood this. The importance of diet was emphasized in *Huangdi Neijing (Yellow Emperor's Classic of Internal Medicine)*: "The five kinds of grains are the mainstay. The five kinds of fruits are to assist. The five animals are to increase. The five kinds of vegetables are to replenish. When the Qi and flavor is right, eat it to supplement the essense and Qi." It means man's diet must be cereals-based, the others are only there to assist and supplement.

EAT FOODS OF DIFFERENT COLORS.

The Alzheimer's Association suggests that most adults should be able to consume around 2,500 calories a day. Fewer calories are needed if people are older or less active. Men should have some 250 grams of unrefined or processed carbohydrates a day, while women should have around 190 grams of unrefined carbohydrates a day.

Most calorie intake should be less-refined, less-processed foods with a low glycemic load (low GI). Intake of protein should be about 100 grams each day. It seems to be beneficial to eat less red meat and eat more fish and high-quality natural cheese and yogurt to obtain the daily quota of protein. Forty grams of fiber is required each day, acquired by consuming fruit (especially berries), vegetables (especially beans), and whole grains.

A healthy diet should include fat. About 67 grams each day in a ratio of 1:2:1 of saturated to monounsaturated to polyunsaturated fat is advisable.

ANTIOXIDANTS PROTECT CELLS FROM DAMAGE

Studies have shown that high intake of saturated fat and cholesterol clogs the arteries and is associated with higher risk for dementia. However, HDL (or "good") cholesterol may help protect brain cells. Moreover, recent research suggests that it is the oxidation of LDL, the "bad" cholesterol, when accumulated in the walls of damaged arteries that causes the thickening that leads to reduced blood flow and blockage.

Reduction of saturated fats from daily meals should be offset by ensuring intake of adequate essential fatty acids, especially the omega-3s. Polyunsaturated omega fatty acids found in fish, some seeds and fruits are associated with a lower risk of dementia. Cold-water fish contain beneficial omega-3 fatty acids: halibut, mackerel, salmon, trout, and tuna. Canned fish is a real alternative, or fish oil capsules can be taken each day.

A diet that is low in saturated fat and high in fiber enhances general well-being. A diet high in fiber from whole grain cereals and vegetables aids in digestion and ensures a healthy digestive tract and proper absorption of nutrients. In some cases, especially as we grow older, prebiotics, like natural yogurt, and probiotics can be helpful to maintain gut health and improve absorption of nutrients.

CHRONIC INFLAMMATION DAMAGES THE BODY

According to the Alzheimer's Association, the best way to obtain all the essential daily supply of vitamins, minerals, and micronutrients is by eating fresh foods with lots of whole grain cereals, fruits and vegetables. To get maximum natural protection against age-related diseases (including cardiovascular disease, cancer, and neurodegenerative disease), as well as against environmental toxicity, we should eat foods of different colors, including a variety of cereals, fruits, vegetables, and fungi (mushrooms), especially brown or wild rice, oats, berries, tomatoes, orange and yellow fruits, and dark leafy greens.

Some foods are considered to be protective, with current research suggesting they may reduce the risk of heart disease and stroke and appear to protect brain cells.

Chronic inflammation seems to be one of the main causes of many serious illnesses, including heart disease, many cancers, and dementia. The inflammatory processes are essential in dealing with acute injury or infection by stimulating immune activity.

SUPPLEMENTS ARE IMPORTANT FOR A HEALTHY DIET.

However, when inflammation persists or serves no purpose, it damages the body and causes illness. Poor diet, stress, lack of exercise, genetic predisposition, and exposure to toxins (like secondhand tobacco smoke) can all contribute to chronic inflammation. The best strategy for reducing long-term chronic inflammation is to include ample vitamins, minerals, essential fatty acids, dietary fiber, and protective plant nutrients.

Apart from chronic inflammation, it is thought that oxidative stress resulting in free radicals damage plays a part in people getting dementia. Indeed, evidence from numerous studies indicates that people with dementia have depleted levels of antioxidants in their brains.

Antioxidants are substances that protect cells from the oxidative damage caused by free radicals (unstable molecules made by the process of oxidation during normal metabolism). Antioxidants found in food are important for good health as they "mop up" free radicals that otherwise do so much harm to the body. The body also produces enzymes (longer-acting antioxidants) that act to neutralize the action of free radicals. These enzymes require vitamins (A, C, and E, short-acting antioxidants) and minerals (cofactors) such as selenium, iron, copper, zinc, and manganese to work most effectively.

MULTI-MINERALS ARE IMPORTANT

Fruits and vegetables have naturally occurring antioxidants. Antioxidants inhibit oxidation in the body, by removing free radicals which could otherwise cause cell damage.

Antioxidants include beta-carotene, lycopene, vitamins A, C, and E, and other natural and manufactured substances. In general, many spices and herbs and dark-skinned fruits and vegetables have the highest levels of naturally occurring antioxidant levels. These vegetables include kale, spinach, brussels sprouts, alfalfa sprouts, broccoli, beets, red bell pepper, onion, corn, and eggplant.

Fruits with high antioxidant levels include acai berries and cranberries, prunes, raisins, blueberries, blackberries, strawberries, raspberries, plums, oranges, red grapes, and cherries. Research studies have indicated that naturally occurring chemicals in red- or purple-skinned fruits, peanuts and in red wine act as antioxidants. The antioxidants in red wine are called flavonoids and come from the fermentation of the grape skins.

FRESH FOOD CONTAINS BENEFICIAL, LIVE ENZYMES

However, an inadequate dietary intake of trace minerals may compromise the effectiveness of these antioxidant defense mechanisms, as the absorption of important trace minerals tends to decrease with aging. Therefore a supplement of multi-minerals may be an important component of a good diet and may be essential to get any benefit from taking antioxidants.

Scientific studies have shown that a diet that includes daily intake of fruit and vegetables at adequate levels improves health and reduces mortality due to cardiovascular disease. A recent European study following over 25,000 people over thirteen years showed that eating around 500 grams of fruit and vegetables a day reduced mortality by 10 percent.

Food that is bought fresh and more closely resembles food in its most natural state is nutrient-dense and contains lots of beneficial, live enzymes. Fresh food and naturally derived supplements provide readily absorbed antioxidants such as carotenes, flavonoids, zinc, and selenium, which are considered to be protective of degenerative disease, while refined, processed, takeout food that is full of preservatives is not fresh food and is often not nutritious.

A diet that contains some protein for breakfast and lunch and includes lecithin and ground flaxseed, such as a salad with tuna or salmon, may improve brain function and alertness. Later in the day, meals containing high proportions of carbohydrates such as pasta (made from whole grains) with some protein would be most ideal, as they help people relax and have more restful sleep.

THERE NATURALLY OCCURRING ANTIOXIDANTS.

On the other hand, while vitamins, minerals, and antioxidants occur naturally, concentrated formulations may make them more convenient to take and ensure we get optimum amounts each day. Vitamins A, C, and E are not produced by the body and are required daily. Vitamin C is not made in our bodies and must be taken in through foods and supplements. It is readily absorbed and is nontoxic. It is also important in the action of enzymes, which also act as antioxidants among other vital functions. Vitamin C is most commonly used to treat the common cold. As a powerful antioxidant, it boosts the immune system and is used to increase the absorption of iron from food. Iron in the blood carries oxygen around the body, including the brain. It is therefore thought to provide some benefits by increasing oxygen availability and may be useful for improving brain function, including dementia and depression.

A HEALTHY DIET SHOULD INCLUDE FAT.

While it is available in many foods and vitamin E deficiency is very rare, vitamin E is an antioxidant and needs to be consumed daily at adequate levels to be protective.

Natural food sources containing vitamin E include vegetable oils, cereals, meat, poultry, eggs, fruits, vegetables, wheat-germ oil, sunflower and safflower oil, nuts and seeds (almonds, sunflower seeds, peanuts, hazelnuts), and green vegetables, including broccoli and spinach. When mixed with a little healthy fat and eating green vegetables, the absorption of vitamin E is maximized.

Research showed that those with the highest amounts of vitamin E in their diet (from food, not supplements, in this study) have a significantly lower risk of developing and a better chance of controlling symptoms of chronic disease. If dietary intake is not adequate, taking vitamin E as a supplement may prevent diseases of the brain, muscles, and nervous system, including Alzheimer's disease and other dementias.

There are many other naturally occurring antioxidants: vitamin-like substances such as bioflavonoids, co-enzyme Q-10, and alpha-lipoic acid, found in abundance in many plants. It is widely accepted that antioxidants are required for the proper function of many organs and chemical reactions in the body. They help provide energy to cells, as well as neutralize free radicals that promote degenerative processes.

MAINTAINING GOOD NUTRITION IS CHALLENGING.

While co-enzyme Q-10 occurs throughout the body and is found in some meats and fish and while alpha-lipoic acid is found in yeast, liver, kidney, spinach, broccoli, and potatoes, they become depleted as we age. They can also be obtained as dietary supplements.

Alpha-lipoic acid is approved in some European countries for treatment of diabetes and nerve-related symptoms of diabetes, and co-enzyme Q-10 is very popular in Japan and some parts of Europe. Some people use antioxidants to combat memory loss, chronic fatigue syndrome (CFS), HIV/AIDS, cancer, and diseases of the heart and blood.

Alpha-lipoic acid is also used to treat eye-related disorders, such as damage to the retina, cataracts, and glaucoma, and is utilized in the body to break down carbohydrates and to make energy for the other organs in the body.

ANTIOXIDANTS MIGHT BE HELPFUL IN LIVER DISEASES.

As with other antioxidants, coenzyme Q-10 and alpha-lipoic acid seem to help prevent certain kinds of cell damage in the body and also restore vitamin levels such as of vitamin E and vitamin C. There is some evidence that alpha-lipoic acid can improve the function and conduction of neurons, although no studies have conclusively proved these changes are due to the action of these substances.

In some forms antiuoxidants are often not well-absorbed, metabolize quite quickly, and pass out of our bodies before they can do much. On the other hand, good-quality products do seem to boost measures of antioxidant activity, especially in the gut.

One source of antioxidants that seems to deliver them in high quantities and has been shown to have significant beneficial effects comes from the berries of a South American palm tree (acai). A randomized, controlled placebo trial showed impressive increases in blood levels of antioxidants and reductions in oxidative stress factors when taken compared to a group who did not take it.

THE QUALITY OF FOOD HAS DECLINED.

In further studies these berry extracts produced significant reductions in pain and increased ease of movement among arthritis sufferers by reducing inflammation of joints. These were related to measurable reductions in sugar, insulin, and total cholesterol levels, which are markers for cardiovascular disease.

Inadequate levels of vitamins B6, B9 (folic acid), and B12 are implicated in an increase in homocysteines. High levels of these chemicals may pose a greater risk to health than cholesterol, and both have been shown to raise the risk of cardiovascular and Alzheimer's disease.

Recent randomized controlled studies have shown that folate and other vitamin B supplements may slow cognitive decline in older people and that this may be related to lowered homocysteine levels. Hence, adequate nutrient intake, including the vitamin B group, may be useful in preventing memory loss and Alzheimer's disease.

More specifically, vitamin B12 deficiency is thought to be a cause of dementia. As people age they absorb vitamins less efficiently from their food. As B12 is found in meat, fish, poultry, eggs, and dairy products, those with low intake, especially vegetarians, need to take B12 as a supplement. Early symptoms of B12 deficiency are confusion, apathy, irritability, and slowness, which can also be mistaken for depression.

NUTRIENTS ARE IN PULP, SKINS, AND SEED KERNELS.

Flaxseed is a good source of dietary fiber and omega-3 fatty acids and may complement the use of probiotics, as it has been used for many conditions related to the gastrointestinal tract, including ongoing constipation, colon damage due to overuse of laxatives, diarrhea, inflammation of the lining of the large intestine, irritable bowel syndrome, and irritable colon.

However, as indicated above, it may be that large amounts of a wide range of food of these different categories are required to get the nutrients we need. As the soil is depleted of the minerals we need and as food becomes more processed and stored longer, the nutrient value tends to be less than it was only a few years ago.

Moreover, as we age the body becomes less efficient in absorbing essential vitamins and nutrients. Therefore, preparations that have high concentrations of the natural products we need may be helpful if taken daily. This is particularly beneficial if the products include the nutrients contained in the pulp, skins, and seed kernels of the food they are made from—more than if they only contain natural color, flavor, and preservatives derived from the food.

EAT DIETS LOW IN SATURATED FAT AND HIGH IN FIBER.

The best products contain a complete and balanced range of all the vitamins, minerals, and other phytochemicals we need each day for optimal health. For example, the bioflavonoids found in plants seem to improve vitamin C absorption.

Vitamin C strengthens capillary walls, reducing inflammation and decreasing the seepage of blood cells and proteins into the tissues, as well as being a powerful antioxidant in its own right.

Regular supplements of vitamin B complex may be an important factor in preventing stroke; studies involving some 55,000 people showed a 7 percent reduction among those taking vitamin B.

Of some significance is the causal relationship between blood supply to the brain and dementia. Mini-strokes, which mostly go unnoticed, are a major factor in vascular dementia and other forms of dementia, and vitamins E and B may have an important role in preventing these events and preventing disease among those who are vulnerable.

GINKGO BILOBA EXTRACT IMPROVES BLOOD CIRCULATION.

Research has indicated that ginkgo biloba extract from the naturally found herb can improve blood circulation to the brain and reduce damage to cells caused by ultraviolet light; it is therefore used for conditions that seem to be due to reduced blood flow in the brain, especially in older people. These conditions include headaches, ringing in the ears, and vertigo. It is also often used for memory disorders, including Alzheimer's disease. As it seems to improve blood circulation, it might also be useful in helping the brain, eyes, ears, and legs function better.

Independent scientific studies have shown, for example, that consistent intake of nutritional and dietary supplements, coupled with light exercise, showed reductions in weight, for an average loss of 6 kilograms over twelve weeks, with significant improvements in measures of glycemic control (blood sugar levels), cardiovascular risk factors, inflammation, and antioxidant status.

In another study, conducted in conjunction with Boston University, the use of bioflavonoids found in grape-seed extract showed improved microvascular (capillary vein) function in participants, indicating that taking this supplement may reduce cardiovascular risk factors.

AS WE AGE WE ABSORB LESS VITAMINS AND NUTRIENTS.

As we age the ability to absorb nutrients from food may be reduced. This can often occur because of disturbances or poor functioning of the stomach and intestines and kidneys and deficiencies in vitamin D and vitamin B12.

Leaky bowel syndrome is well-recognized among older people, and they often experience regular problems with inflammation and irritation of the bowel, poor appetite, indigestion, discomfort, and diarrhea that can be caused by a buildup of bad bacteria. Some of these problems can be directly related to the side effects of medication, including antibiotics that do not discriminate between healthy bacteria required for healthy digestion and pathogens.

Research has shown that certain bacteria in the bowel may promote inflammation, while others may have a more protective role. The cause of this, in turn, is likely to be the regular use of antibiotics, which tend to not only kill the germs (microorganisms/bacteria) that are making us sick, but also bacteria that live in our digestive system and are necessary for proper breakdown of the food we eat and the absorption of nutrients into the body. These good bacteria also prevent the action of bad bacteria and support our immune system, which fights off disease.

BACTERIA IN THE BOWEL PLAY A PROTECTIVE ROLE.

Probiotics and prebiotics are used in an attempt to reintroduce and nurture protective bacteria in the bowel. They can be taken in capsule form, as a powder, or as drinks (milk or yogurt) and consist of yeast or bacteria. They are considered to be safe by authorities and rarely cause any problems.

There is impressive research evidence to support the use of probiotics in treating acute and infectious diarrhea and preventing antibiotic-associated diarrhea and bowel inflammations such as pouchitis, Crohn's disease, and irritable bowel syndrome, and for preventing relapse in patients with ulcerative colitis.

Since the quality of food has declined and the pace of life causes us to value convenience so much, it seems that nutrient supplements are necessary to sustain good health and to ensure that our body can heal itself. As the best supplements are made from food, it only makes sense for us to make use of them to ensure optimum health. To state the obvious, there are no side effects to eating food! It seems we need to educate many doctors about this commonsense approach to prevention of obesity and chronic diseases such as diabetes and dementia.

> ## PREVENTION INVOLVES MEDICATION, EXERCISE, FOOD, AND NUTRITION.

The next chapter is about lifestyle changes that can improve quality of life for someone with dementia and about adapting a "person-centered" approach to caring for the person. I explain this concept of care in the next chapter and expand on this idea in chapters 12 and 13. For now I want to focus on how to work with the person with dementia to maximize health, including prevention of other chronic diseases that might afflict them. Issues include medication, exercise, food, and nutrition.

Chapter 10

What More Can We Do?

In the last chapter we looked at the importance of prevention implemented well before the onset of chronic age-related diseases. Changes in lifestyle made early enough can have a profound effect on how healthy we are and how well we can live. However, caring for someone with dementia can become very difficult both for you and them. The legal rights of someone with dementia need to be considered; looking after finances can become touchy. I deal with these problems in Chapter 14 of the book.

> A WIDE VARIETY OF DRUGS CAN MAKE SYMPTOMS WORSE.

Despite the inevitable decline in functioning, there are many things we can do to make life easier and to maximize quality of life for everyone. Even at a time when dementia is a reality, lifestyle change can still bring significant benefits. The approach is often referred to as person-centered care. It is a style of caring that also minimizes the stress of the caregiver. It is the system of care that I refer to in chapter 12 when I talk of aged day-care centers and in chapter 13.

As mentioned earlier dementia may be accompanied by a range of symptoms that may or may not be symptoms of the disease. These include depression, loss of appetite, and sleep deprivation, and in some cases, behavioral disturbance and hallucinations. Often medications are prescribed that can be helpful, such as antidepressants. Some medications, in particular for some forms of dementia, may improve a range of symptoms and delay onset; however, a wide variety of drugs can make them worse. That is, certain medications can have a positive effect on our brain functioning, and some that are prescribed to people with dementia should be avoided.

ANTIPSYCHOTICS SHOULD BE USED WITH CAUTION

Many dementia sufferers are medicated using antipsychotics that are thought to reduce anxiety, hallucinations, and aggression. However, not only are some dementias made worse by the use of these drugs, but also research has demonstrated that behavioral problems can be more efficiently managed using person-centered caring strategies, which are described in later chapters. Use of these medicines, even at small doses, can cause particularly severe side effects for those with Lewy body dementia. As there is considerable overlap between types of dementia, those with Alzheimer's disease may have an underlying Lewy body pathology and be similarly affected.

Quite apart from the potential abuse of these drugs to manage people, antipsychotic drugs should be used with caution in people with dementia. They tend to slow responses and may even be the leading cause of the apathy that is so often seen in people with dementia. Surveys of aged-care facilities in Australia show that on average some 30 percent of elderly people with dementia are medicated with antipsychotics. Some facilities use them as management tools, with up to 80 percent of their dementia patients being given them in some facilities with little justification.

ACCURATE DIAGNOSIS SHOULD PRECEDE MEDICATION.

Often elderly people with dementia are treated with anticholinergic medication for incontinence, breathing difficulties, and urinary tract infections. However, most people as they get older experience deficits in the production of acetylcholine (an essential brain-signaling chemical). These medications make that deficit worse, making unwanted side effects more pronounced in those with dementia. Again, caring strategies to reduce the need for medication, such as the bathroom being lit at night and easily seen from the bed, reduce bed-wetting and spoiling. Anticholinergic use should be carefully monitored and used with caution. As a result of the problems thought to be caused by these medications, claims have been made that drugs that reduce acetylcholine levels (anticholinesterase inhibitors) may be beneficial for those in the early stages of dementia. However, trial results have not been impressive, despite early promise. Aricept is one of these drugs that have been given to people with dementia. The most benefit seems to be for those diagnosed early. However, it seems that at best it delays the onset of dementia by only six months.

HEALTHY DIET REDUCES RISK OF HEART DISEASE AND DIABETES.

Other medications that can cause memory loss and confusion include some antidepressants, anticonvulsants, antihistamines, corticosteroids, sedatives, and some narcotic painkillers.

Some authorities warn against synthetic medications and supplements when natural substances either in foods or as extracts are available. For example, natural progesterone and other hormone replacements have been shown to be better, with fewer side effects, than synthetic substitutes.

Moreover, recent studies have shown that women who undergo estrogen or estrogen-progesterone replacement therapy are at increased risk of dementia. In some cases natural products may not be any more effective than easily obtainable drugs. However, as is the case with natural hormone replacements and natural products such as St. John's wort (for depression) or ginkgo biloba (for cardiovascular health), they generally have no serious side effects and do not have problems with interactions with other medications.

DO NOT DISCOUNT THE INCREDIBLE ADVANCES IN MEDICAL SCIENCE

The doctor can check all this out with you, as it is imperative that an accurate diagnosis of the disease is made before any medications are prescribed and that a thorough review of medication is made after diagnosis. A good doctor should also be able to suggest natural products to replace synthetic products, or a referral to a natural health therapist or nutritionist may be helpful.

We must be careful not to discount the incredible advances in medical science and understand that much of our ability to live so much longer is attributable to these advances. Surgical techniques, antibiotics, chemo, and radiotherapy now see miracles performed every day to restore people to health who would have died only a few years ago.

Eating a well-balanced, nutritious diet can also be highly beneficial for your general health and particularly a healthy cardiovascular system. While age and family history (genetics) are risk factors, research suggests that lifestyle factors, including diet and exercise, play a vital role in the prevention of dementia. Good nutrition combined with moderate to heavy exercise can decrease the risk of dementia by some 45 percent.

POORLY NOURISHED PEOPLE GET SICK MORE OFTEN.

Moderate exercise includes house and light outside work (sweeping, hosing the garden), climbing stairs, and sports like swimming, bowling and golf. Being fit has been shown to reduce damage to brain cells, which is related to dementia, and may help fight depression, which also commonly occurs in people with the disease. Exercise should be discussed with the person with dementia; it should be appropriate, and it should be enjoyable. Activities done in groups, like aqua aerobics, garden excursions, and bush walks, can be both beneficial and fun.

It was thought that no special diet was specific for the prevention of dementia, including Alzheimer's disease.

However, with the realization that a healthy diet can benefit other conditions, such as diabetes and heart disease, and as a healthy brain and a healthy heart are very closely related, there may be an indirect impact on prevention of dementia. More importantly we now understand that the fundamental causes of most chronic disease are attributable to the damage to cells from oxidative stress and chronic inflammation.

A DEPRESSED PERSON IS LESS MOTIVATED.

While there have been many claims made for "brain food" to prevent or reverse dementia, the research is not conclusive, although the principles applied to general well-being can be applied here. For example, brain messenger chemicals (acetylcholine, dopamine, serotonin, and glutamate) known as neurotransmitters are essential for healthy brain function. Many are found in many foods such as beans, liver, whole grains, foods rich in chlorophyll, soy, lecithin, and egg yolks. The basic rule is to eat a variety of foods from each food category.

As stated, a healthy diet for the brain is one that reduces the risk of heart disease and diabetes, encourages good blood flow to the brain, and is high in low GI foods and low in salt and cholesterol. Like the heart, the brain needs the right balance of nutrients, including protein and carbohydrates, to function well. A healthy diet is most effective when combined with physical activity, mental activity, and social interaction. Poorly nourished people get sick more often and recover from injury and illness more slowly, and poor nutrition is a major health problem for many older people.

INSOMNIA IS A PROBLEM AS WE GET OLDER.

A proper diet and good-quality supplements enable the body to work more efficiently, provide more energy, enhance the effect of medications, and control weight better for overall good health of the brain and body. A long-term study of 1,500 adults found that those who were obese in middle age were twice as likely to develop dementia in later life and those who also had high cholesterol and high blood pressure had six times the risk of dementia.

Depression and grief, which are prevalent among older people, can result in loss of motivation, and hence, a disinclination to prepare food and eat properly. As intake declines and the food becomes less nutritious, sometimes a vicious cycle can be the result in deficiencies in vital vitamins and minerals and a buildup of toxins in the body and brain. This, in turn, can reduce appetite and lead to sleep disturbance, making the depression worse.

A good intake of fresh foods is an essential component of good health. However, a person with dementia may experience a loss of appetite, develop a craving for sweet foods, forget to eat and drink, and forget how to chew or swallow. They may experience a dry mouth or mouth discomfort, often related to badly fitting false teeth or tooth decay, and food and drink may not be recognized or not considered palatable.

PEOPLE WITH DEMENTIA MAY FORGET TO EAT.

As a result there is a greater risk of being malnourished or lacking certain essential vitamins, minerals, and nutrients as people get older. They may be less likely to prepare food just for themselves, and rely more on snacks like biscuits. Often appetite is diminished with less activity, and they often forget to eat. A person who is depressed is much less motivated to make an effort, which tends to make things worse.

As we age, the vitamins and minerals found in food provide the foundation for the body's defenses against viruses, ailments, and degenerative diseases, However, with a decline in appetite and a reduced ability to break down foods to access these essential elements, a diet that includes supplements of vitamins, minerals, fatty acids, and antioxidants becomes necessary to maintain health and nourish the brain.

Studies indicate that a regular intake of fresh fruit and vegetables is beneficial and reduces mortality by improving cardiovascular function. A study of elderly women showed that those who ate the most green, leafy, and cruciferous vegetables in the group were one to two years younger in mental function than women who ate few of these vegetables.

MODERATE ALCOHOL USE MAY STIMULATE APPETITE.

As mentioned dementia is often accompanied by other problems that contribute to poor functioning that may not be caused by the disease but that might make it worse. Problems being able to sleep are common as we get older, and they are likely to make worse other problems, such as irritability and depression. Melatonin is a naturally occurring hormone in the body and can be made into a pill form. Darkness tends to promote an increase in this hormone and prepares us for sleep, while light causes levels to fall. Some people who have trouble sleeping have low levels of melatonin. Adding melatonin from supplements might help adjust the sleep cycle, assist them to fall asleep, and allow less-disturbed sleep. Some people have used melatonin to treat Alzheimer's disease. However, there is no evidence to show it can directly alleviate any symptoms apart from improving sleep.

VITAMIN D IS MAINLY REPLENISHED BY SUNLIGHT.

It is very common for older people to suffer from calcium and vitamin D deficiency, leading to problems with the chemical balance in the blood and regulation of nerve signals, brittle bones, and skin conditions. Anyone over sixty-five is at risk of being calcium- and vitamin D-deficient and may be vulnerable to the health consequences. Calcium deficiency is countered by the body using up reserves from the bones, which leads to osteoporosis (weakening of the bones, leading to fractures in the elderly). While vitamin D is available in some foods, it is mainly replenished by exposure to sunlight. Even in sunny climates, up to 40 percent of older people are vulnerable and don't have enough vitamin D in their systems as they don't venture into the sunlight as often and may have trouble metabolizing it. Vitamin D supplements are often necessary for people who do not have enough time in sunshine or who live in colder climates.

Maintaining good nutrition presents extra challenges for people with dementia. A decline in quality of life can be slowed even at later stages of the disease, with diet and nutrition playing an important role in being healthy and feeling good. However, encouraging your loved one to eat regularly can often be a real concern for caregivers.

People with dementia may forget to eat. Setting an alarm clock or receiving a phone call may be useful reminders of mealtimes. Finger foods and fruit can be left out where they can be easily seen.

ALCOHOL CAN CONTRIBUTE TO FEELINGS OF DEPRESSION.

Meals should be shared whenever possible, with an occasional visit to your favorite restaurant to encourage your loved one to eat. In addition to sitting for a while and sharing some food and a chat, family and friends can help by preparing meals and freezing large quantities of meal-size amounts of food, as well as by stocking up on healthy snacks such as yogurt, cheese, or dried fruit that do not need preparation or cooking and buying frozen vegetables from the supermarket. At other times, agencies and government-funded home support programs can provide assistance with meal preparation and serving and discretely encourage regular eating (see EACHD, p. 97). Not only will diet and physical health be improved, but also these are opportunities for social interaction to nourish the soul and enhance emotional well-being that will outlast the memory of the occasion.

FUNCTIONING CAN BE IMPROVED BY MODIFYING TASKS.

Moderate alcohol use may stimulate the appetite and add to the enjoyment of a meal. However, too much alcohol can replace food, and people can run the risk of becoming malnourished as alcohol has no nutritional value. Being a depressant, alcohol can also contribute to feelings of depression, which can impact on motivation and appetite. It may be difficult for a person with dementia who is a heavy drinker to change his or her drinking habits. Cutting down alcohol consumption by ensuring he or she eats well, discouraging drinking on an empty stomach, and offering nonalcoholic and watered-down alcoholic drinks may be successful.

As well as diet and exercise, socialization, a secure environment, and sensory stimulation have all shown benefits in terms of creating positive feelings and improving health and quality of life. However, decline in functioning is inevitable. Functioning can be improved by modifying tasks or the environment or by coming up with workable strategies to perform these functions.

The consequence of this realization as the disease progresses is that the aim of caregivers, with the involvement of the person with dementia, is to develop compensatory strategies to improve quality of life and to improve independence for as long as possible.

ABILITIES OF THE PERSON WITH DEMENTIA ARE IMPORTANT.

In caring for someone with dementia, the aim is to improve or maximize function and to focus on capacities that are intact or can be compensated for, rather than impairment and symptoms. In practical terms that means providing aids to maintain functionality and maximize safety by improving capacity to self-manage personal, domestic, community, and social activities. Improved functioning can be achieved by modifying tasks or the environment or by coming up with workable strategies to perform these functions. It tends to enhance a positive disposition and helps to maintain a sense of autonomy and self-respect.

Strategies and modifications should be worked out together as a family, and training and practice in the person's environment will ensure that the changes are effective in the context of the practical realities of the person's strengths and weaknesses, their situation, and their needs.

It cannot be overemphasized that the abilities of the person with dementia need to be taken into account. Not only will the tendency for us to take over rob them of their dignity, but it may well mean we carry a burden unnecessarily that can become too much in time.

PEOPLE MIGHT REJECT HELP IF THEY THINK THEY ARE BEING DISPLACED.

To make matters worse, we could inadvertently set up an expectation that we will do certain things, even though it may not be necessary, at least in the short term. An unhealthy dependency might grow that is not in anyone's interests.

Taking over may also mean we are not providing opportunities for activities or tasks that are meaningful. Planning strategies should be an opportunity for learning and promoting a sense of achievement. Verbal cues might be sufficient to do routine things without having to fully supervise or perform the task for the person with dementia and yet still ensure good health and safety. Tasks that can be minimally supervised can be established over time, maximizing independence even though they may not be sustainable after a period as the person's condition inevitably declines. People who might reject help if they think they are being displaced or made to feel useless may be amenable to being gently reminded or coaxed to do daily tasks, such as hygiene, in their own time.

CALENDARS AND A NOTEBOOK CAN BE HELPFUL.

The type of assistance should be based on an assessment of the performance of the person with dementia when doing a particular task, and strategies and modifications need to be evaluated. Sometimes finding an easier way of doing something might be helpful. For example, the use of blister packs or medication dispensers that check off the date or time medication should be taken can ease the burden of worrying whether too much or too little has been taken, simplifying instructions and removing unnecessary information.

Some tasks may be avoided, such as having a set menu and having groceries or meals delivered. The use of calendars and a notebook to remind the person of important appointments or routine tasks can be useful in the early stages. Instructions or directions should be given one at a time, rather than a number together, as it becomes hard to hold a whole lot of things in their heads at one time, let alone juggle them about. Instructions to do things, like recipes and other daily tasks, can be rewritten so one thing can be accomplished at a time and nonvital steps removed.

DO NOT DISREGARD VAGUE OR UNREALISTIC IDEAS.

It is sometimes helpful to have photographs of what is to be done at each stage. Verbal instructions could be given in a sequential way as one element of a task is completed and to ensure the time between an instruction and when it needs to be done is minimized. Not only does this give a jog to the memory; it also minimizes confusion about the way to do something, and it also builds confidence and encourages independence.

In developing strategies to accomplish tasks, it is crucial to include the person with dementia and to account for his or her abilities, limitations, and needs. When language and communication have been compromised, the person's preferences can be difficult to accurately determine. It may, therefore, be difficult for them to provide any precise idea as to what they want to accomplish and how.

Often goals may be expressed as vague wishes that may be quite unrealistic given the level of impairment.

However, it is important not to disregard these ideas or to be put off by difficulties in making clear their meaning. Better to use them as a starting point to develop strategies to achieve goals that are realistic and achievable. Doing a task that may require sustained effort and attention may not be possible.

DISTRACTIONS CAN WORK WELL SOMETIMES

A lack of initiative may indicate how daunting a task may appear, not laziness, even when it is an activity they have voiced a preference for. Breaking tasks up into manageable chunks not only allows the person to maintain concentration, but also reduces fatigue and stress. At these times reducing the number of distractions or interruptions, like reducing noise, visual distractions like a TV, or the demands of others, is important in allowing the person to focus and to maximize attention.

Frustration and getting upset is not uncommon when trying to reach goals that are difficult or not regarded as important or that are thought to be imposed or intrusive. To push the point can be a wrong move, and a simple strategy to defuse a nasty situation is to divert their attention toward something entirely different—so distractions can work well if it all gets to be too much. This may sound manipulative; however, three things should be kept in mind.

First, a person with dementia can tend to become fixated on an issue or problem that is not immediately resolvable or is causing them to get distressed, so no good can come from keeping it going. Second, they may have a very real objection or a good point that needs to be heeded and worked into any new strategy. Third, they may just be exhausted and need a break.

THE ENVIRONMENTAL CHANGE CAN BE QUICK AND SAFE.

An obvious approach is to look at how the environment can be changed to achieve goals easily and safely. Things such as: electronic devices that are simple to operate or retain analogue controls, such as a radio that is locked onto their favorite station or a TV guide that is written out so favorite shows are readily noted and not missed; chairs that are not too hard to get out of; simplifying a wardrobe of clothes so choices are fewer and less confusing; bathtubs or showers that have a step where the ground is lower than the bottom of the bath or shower; nonslip mats and surfaces; and signs that are easily read.

The aim should be to make appropriate changes to the nature of tasks and the way they are done and to the environment to maximize functioning, independence, and safety.

Safety tends to become a major concern, especially when there is the tendency to forget to turn off heaters or stoves or to fall and not be able to get help.

QUALITY OF LIFE FOR CAREGIVERS IS RELATED TO HIGHER QUALITY OF LIFE FOR THE PERSON WITH DEMENTIA

Not remembering to eat or wash can constitute preventable causes of deterioration in health or disease. Signs on things have been found to be helpful, especially when there is a photograph or diagram illustrating what needs to be done; and timers can be used to signal mealtimes and other important daily activities. Automatic shutoff devices can be fitted; and water, smoke, or personal alarms are available.

All this can seem overwhelming, and you may therefore seek professional support to intervene to improve symptoms and functioning, to find the resources you need, and to implement change in a helpful way. The next chapter deals with the role of health professionals in assisting in the 444, management, and treatment of dementia. As the quality of life for caregivers is related to higher quality of life for the person with dementia, so quality of life for the individual with dementia is related to improved quality of life for the caregiver. At the heart of this is effective communication and respect for each other, with a focus on maximizing functioning.

Chapter 11

What Can Health Professionals Do?

The primary role of health professionals is to provide a thorough and accurate assessment and to provide a treatment plan and strategies with your and your loved one's needs and preferences as the major concern. Assessment focuses on the person's strengths or those abilities that are intact and can be built on to maximize functioning.

> PEOPLE WITH DEMENTIA CAN HAVE PROBLEM WITH TRUST.

This chapter describes the process of assessment and the types of strategies that can be developed. Some of these are described above in the chapter on what you can do. However, sometimes a professional can be helpful in providing a program that is based on a realistic appraisal of what is possible as well as the limitations of what is achievable now and later when symptoms become more severe; these considerations should be incorporated into any plan.

At the heart of assessment is the capacity to communicate, to enable the taking of a detailed history, to ensure instructions to complete tests are understood, and to understand the subjective world of the person with dementia. However, people with dementia often have problems with trust and view the health professional with suspicion, especially if they associate assessment with admission to an old person's home. They often have problems with language and understanding complex instructions or explanations as the brain disease progresses.

VERBAL AND NONVERBAL AFFIRMATIONS ARE REASSURING.

The health practitioner should be aware of these deficits and find a way of communicating that takes this into account. Providing instructions one at a time, minimizing distractions, taking time to account for fatigue and loss of concentration, and writing or using models or illustrations to provide clear explanations and to convey meaning about the disease or the treatment plan are all techniques to ensure the person understands. More importantly they demonstrate a respectful concern for the person and respects their right to know and to be a part of the process. These are the factors upon which rapport is developed, and this is the most important component in gaining trust and the cooperation of the person with dementia.

People with dementia often complain about people, including health professionals, who shout, talk as if they are not there, and do not bother to explain what is happening. They can become annoyed when they are treated as if they are stupid, or when others do not listen to what they are trying to say, pretend to understand when it is obvious they do not, rush through explanations, and do not take account of their fears and anxiety.

TESTS INCLUDE BLOOD ANALYSIS AND BRAIN SCANS

Reassurance can be achieved by maintaining as much contact with the person as possible by verbal and nonverbal affirmations, indicating that they have been heard. Eye contact, facial responsiveness, including the person in the planning of treatment, and using diagrams or models to illustrate explanations or specific suggestions for when to take medication are helpful. Sometimes physical contact may be appropriate to develop rapport and instill confidence.

Assessment requires the input of a number of health professionals. Most importantly is the knowledge and expertise of a specialist doctor who works with older people. These people are known as geriatric physicians, and they are familiar with the signs and symptoms indicative of dementia in the early and later stages. The geriatric physician will take a detailed history, including that of the extended family. They will use structured interviewing techniques aided by instruments such as the MMSE or the NUCOG to make a provisional diagnosis. They will also do a physical examination and order a range of tests. These tests include blood analysis and brain scans to treat associated problems such as high blood pressure or to rule out other problems such as infections, tumors, chemical imbalances, or vascular problems like reductions in blood flow to parts of the brain.

A NEUROPSYCHOLOGIST CAN WORK WITH THE DOCTOR.

A geriatrics doctor will look at physical factors such as disease or illness, to prescribe medication, and to devise a treatment plan, which may include psychological therapy.

At the same time, these professionals need objective information about specific deficits in brain function, whether it is memory, thinking, or judgment. They also need to know to what extent each of these domains of brain functioning are affected and to understand those abilities that are intact. A neuroscientist or neuropsychologist is trained to test for these and to work closely with the geriatrician.

Neuropsychological testing has developed over many years to now allow us to accurately differentiate between and to determine the cause of a range of cognitive or mental impairments. Neuroscientists and neuropsychologists can draw inferences from scores on a range of tests to pinpoint existence and severity of impairment, the part of the brain that is affected, the behavioral consequences, the course of the disease, and the sort of treatments that might be useful.

WE NEED TO TEST FOR PSYCHOLOGICAL PROBLEMS

Touch-screen computer testing allows us to quickly check a range of cognitive abilities, before fatigue becomes an important factor, and to compare results with those of thousands of people of the same age, education level, and gender. We can then provide some idea if any changes are reasonable for the person's age or, if they are not, determine the part of the brain that is affected, the cause, the behavioral consequences, and possible environmental factors.

In addition, we need to test for psychological problems to try to understand if these are factors in making the symptoms of dementia worse or if they are a consequence of degenerative disease. Psychological tests have been developed to make it easier for older people to complete these accurately.

Of equal importance is to get a very good idea about what is happening in the life of the person with dementia.

We need to learn about their lifestyle choices and habits, and we need to learn about their history and if other family members have suffered from various illnesses, as sometimes these are genetically linked.

We need to learn about their present relationships and what stresses there are in their lives. All these can be risk factors and are also essential in making some sense of what is happening and determining whether they are suffering from some form of dementia or not and the extent that other factors are making things better or worse.

> ### PEOPLE WITH DEMENTIA ARE OFTEN RELUCTANT TO SEE HEALTH PROFESSIONALS.

Professionals are trained to produce an accurate testing of the patient's mental health. They are also trained to be attentive to their needs and to provide feedback that may be helpful for the professional to make the best decisions for your loved ones.

Some of the essential techniques in communication and development of rapport mean that the person with dementia (and also you) feel that their involvement in the consultation process from the beginning is valued. This involves the health professional making time to adequately establish the relationship, unravel the history, assess communication levels, make a thorough assessment and diagnosis, and provide clear explanations and instructions. This may also involve being prepared to terminate the session early if it becomes apparent that the person is finding it difficult to cope because of anxiety or fatigue. It may be necessary to reschedule a few shorter consultations.

> **TESTS CHECK IF FUNCTIONING IS IN THE NORMAL RANGE.**

At the first interview, the professional should introduce himself or herself to the person first, rather than the family, using respectful terms and asking for permission to greet them by their first name. They may then request the person to introduce their family or caregivers and ask if they would like them to be present during the interview.

Having used this time to gauge the level of communication, it is necessary for the health professional to proceed with care to ensure these first impressions are accurate. The health professional might ask them if they mind if they address some questions to you or the others present if it is believed that the patient does not have sufficient cognitive capacity or verbal skills to ensure an accurate history and symptoms is attainable.

When speaking to the person with dementia, to maximize their understanding and accuracy of the information obtained and also to demonstrate concern for their interests, several techniques are recommended.

Firstly, use simple, appropriate, and clear language, avoiding jargon, asking if there are any questions and waiting for a response at regular intervals. Diagrams and pictures, concrete examples and similes, as well as signs and gestures illustrating the information, can make meaning plainer. To reinforce the message, repetition, frequent checks that everyone understands, and clarification of answers will ensure that everyone is satisfied with the advice given.

> ## THE PERSON WITH DEMENTIA SHOULD FEEL VALUED.

Frequent referral back to the family and caregivers by the health professional to ensure their inclusion in the consultation is also important. Their feelings need to be considered, and to ignore their input or questions can be distressing for them. This includes taking the time to allow others to translate if older relatives cannot understand English very well. Often relatives have a significant influence on the decisions that are made, so their involvement and understanding can be crucial to obtaining the best outcome.

Often those with dementia are reluctant to see health professionals for a number of reasons, and fear of finding out the worst can be an important factor in not taking early action. Information these days is often sourced from electronic media, including the Internet. At the end of this book, I have included the web addresses of a number of organizations that can provide a range of helpful information and assistance.

RESULTS CAN BE TAKEN TO YOUR DOCTOR.

On the website www.mindcheck.com.au, you will find some valuable information. To allow you to get some idea of what is happening before going to your doctor and to provide some incentive for the person with dementia to act to make an appointment, I have developed an online test comprising eighty-six carefully selected questions that cover a range of issues that are very important in helping make an accurate assessment if you or your relative has some of the early signs of dementia. Many questions relate to problems that cause dementia-like symptoms that are not dementia and that are treatable. We can also determine with some accuracy if scores are in line with the normal aging process.

The areas examined include language, memory, thinking and problem solving, orientation or visual/spatial abilities, depression, substance abuse, head injury, and low-and high-level functioning. The test also includes some questions on family history, recent traumatic or stressful events, recent operations or general anesthetics, and if changes have occurred suddenly or gradually.

Each of the nine areas that are examined are scored to indicate whether the score is within the normal range, whether the score may indicate some early problems or what we call mild cognitive impairment, or if something more serious is occurring.

DIAGNOSING DEMENTIA IS A COMPLEX PROBLEM.

The results provide an explanation of the significance of each of the issues we examine, and then a written response is provided that is specific to the person's performance.

Some of the answers may seem complicated. However, they are designed to be printed out for the doctor to analyze, or we can provide further and more detailed explanations.

Diagnosing dementia is a complex problem, mainly because many symptoms can be other things that look like dementia and need to be ruled out. Having the test can avoid needless worrying, or an individual can seek early treatment and reap enormous benefits from doing something about it without delay.

The results can indicate if a person has a particular type of dementia. If it seems that there has been quite a sudden change, this may indicate vascular dementia, as reduction or cessation in the flow of blood to certain parts of the brain can cause certain sorts of problems.

OFTEN FEAR OF THE UNKNOWN PREVENTS ACTION.

Some signs become evident early, like loss of orientation, not knowing where you are, forgetting important things like turning off stoves or heaters or repeating the same things, or other problems like loss of feeling or movement on one side of the body or blacking out.

If this is happening to the person you are worried about, they should go to an emergency department of the local hospital. It may indicate a stroke that should be treated immediately to prevent further brain damage. If symptoms are mild and have been complained about for some time, you should go to the GP and get a referral to see a specialist to have a full assessment, including blood tests and brain scans to test if they have developed a tumor or have had a mild stroke, suffered a head injury, or have other problems that affect a particular part of the brain. This is most likely in people under fifty-five, as dementia and Alzheimer's disease are rare for younger people, although people seem to be getting them younger these days.

It is also possible that someone who is younger and who shows signs of failing intellect has developed motor neuron disease, which can affect thinking and memory and is not just confined to impairment of movement.

> **THERE COMES A TIME WHEN WE CANNOT COPE ANYMORE.**

If the brain scan does not show any of these signs, then it is possible that they have developed a type of dementia like Alzheimer's disease. Perhaps you have only just started to notice more severe symptoms, as it is normally quite a gradual process.

Seeking professional advice as early as possible can help alleviate a lot of fears. Often it is fear of the unknown that prevents action, and taking the step to find out can put you and your loved one in control again and take away the fear. Doing something and not being afraid can make everyone feel a lot better.

Despite our best efforts, there comes a time when we cannot cope anymore, and some difficult decisions need to be made. Hopefully, most difficulties have been thought through with the inclusion of the person with dementia at an early stage and with your health professional before symptoms preclude this possibility. The next chapter deals with many of these questions and offers some practical solutions.

Chapter 12

What to Do When We Can't Cope Anymore: Support Services and New Strategies

Dementia or Alzheimer's disease is progressive, meaning that it gets worse over time, with memory failing to the point where loved ones are not recognized. Other problems with language, orientation, thinking logically, becoming aggressive or angry, and behaviors that are troubling develop in time.

> WE CAN FIND IT HARD TO ACCEPT WE CANNOT COPE.

While it is possible for us, as partners, brothers, sisters, or children, to look after an individual with dementia for some years in many cases, there comes a time when this is too much, and we find ourselves out of our depth. A realization that this stage has come is very distressing and hard to accept, making us feel that we have failed or let our loved ones down when they are so vulnerable. And it is often a time when families can find themselves arguing about who should take responsibility, with feelings of shame and guilt running high. This disagreement can revolve around a number of issues: "Why can't the caregiver keep caring?" "Isn't babysitting an easy option compared to other responsibilities we have?" "We promised we would look after them and not let them end up in a home!" "Who will pay?" "What about our inheritance?" "It looks like we don't care and we are just dumping them!"

Often people who are removed from the day-to-day struggle of supporting someone in the middle or later stages of dementia do not appreciate the physical and psychological toll this can bring.

THE CAREGIVER IS OFTEN THE WIFE OR DAUGHTER.

Caring full-time means that you face the realization that the one you loved is no longer present; that they are now different; they can become angry or apathetic, argumentative or emotionally hurt, a danger to themselves and those around them, with the constant fear and responsibility of them wandering off and becoming lost.

Most of all the constant vigilance means that your life is on hold and other responsibilities, obligations, and pleasures foregone. Your partner, friends, and children all have to be denied at least some of your time as the caregiver.

Sometimes it is possible to enlist others to take their turn, but sometimes that is impossible. The role most often seems to fall on the female partner or the daughter, and sons and brothers tend not to see it as their role, especially if they are contributing money and other resources.

Funding for retirement and care is an emerging problem for the community as the population gets older. People's retirement expectations have changed dramatically over the past century, but their savings have not kept pace as the elderly are working less and spending more time in retirement than ever before.

RELIEF IS PROVIDED BY GOVERNMENT PROGRAMS.

At the turn of the century before last, only about half of all Australians reached the age of sixty-five. Now they expect to spend twenty years in retirement after reaching the old-age milestone. To do so they will need to have significant savings or a high retirement income to maintain their standard of living in retirement.

In Australia this concern prompted the government to increase the superannuation guarantee from 9 percent to 12 percent. Such a move would boost the average superannuation balance, but there would still be a gender gap between men and women, and the increase in super contributions would also reduce the government's age-pension burden by 2.3 percent. However, a budget crisis looms as in most countries as the population ages and fewer people are working. There is talk of increasing the pension or retirement age to seventy.

Some relief can be provided by government-funded programs. In some countries, at the local level, day-care programs are offered that are, at best, enriching and have the capacity to improve function and quality of life. At the least they keep people safe while caregivers have time to do the shopping, see to others' needs, and find some time for themselves.

RESPITE CARE GIVES CAREGIVERS THE ENERGY TO GO ON.

Funding is also available for having in-home care from someone to come to do the housework, shopping, or maintenance. In-home nursing is also available. Most programs are limited and provide some relief, especially for elderly spouses who are the primary caregivers. Respite care is available for a limited number of days each year so that caregivers can regroup and find the energy to go on.

Some families therefore turn to government or privately funded support in the home. These services are sometimes available from weekly visits to do shopping, cleaning, cooking, gardening, maintenance, or just keeping the person with dementia occupied, to full-time twenty-four-hour nursing care from professional services, which can cost up to $800 per day, to having an untrained person act as a caregiver, for which payment may be offset by free rent.

In Australia the Commonwealth government provides a range of community care services aimed to help people with a disability live independently in their own homes and maximize quality of life for as long as possible.

PEOPLE CAN LIVE LONGER IN THEIR OWN HOMES

The implementation of these schemes has had a dramatic impact on numbers of people needing residential care and have had a major impact on national expenditure on aged care. More importantly they have allowed people to live longer independently in their own homes and consequently improved their quality of life.

The following information is extracted from the Commonwealth Department of Health and Ageing website. Much more detailed information can be accessed by contacting the government department. Contact details can be found in the Resources section of this book on page 184.

Information for people in need and for others who provide community care services, including respite is provided by Commonwealth Respite and Carelink Centres. Such centers provide free and confidential information on respite community aged care, disability, and other support services available locally, interstate, or anywhere within Australia.

The centers are also able to put people in touch with aged-care assessment teams who can determine who qualifies for assistance for a range of services so that they can continue living in their own home or enter an aged-care home such as a nursing home or hostel.

> **AGED-CARE ASSESSMENT TEAMS HELP WITH SERVICES.**

Other services provide free information and assess the needs of older people and help them get to the services that can assist them to remain living at home, while respite services are available to support to older people, people with a disability, and their caregivers who may need a break or need some extra care for a short period.

Community Care Services involves two programs: Community Aged Care Packages (CACPs) provide low-level aged care in the home for people needing personal care, domestic assistance, and similar services. Extended Aged Care at Home Packages (EACH) provide high-level care to people who need more help than a Community Aged Care Package can provide.

Specific programs for people with dementia include the Extended Aged Care at Home Dementia (EACHD) packages, which provide high-level care to people at the highest end of the community care continuum who experience difficulties in their daily life because of behavioral and psychological symptoms associated with dementia.

> PRIVATE AGED-CARE SERVICES PROVIDE ASSISTANCE UP TO TWENTY-FOUR HOURS A DAY.

Psychogeriatric Care Units (PGUs) help and train staff in aged-care homes and family caregivers to look after people with dementia and challenging behaviors, while The National Continence Management Strategy has introduced a range of measures to help people deal with incontinence.

In addition, the Day Therapy Center Program is funded to provide a range of service to older people and people with disabilities, and the Assistance with Care and Housing for the Aged (ACHA) program provides assistance for financially disadvantaged older people who are renting or who are homeless to access both community care and accommodation.

The Commonwealth government-funded Retirement Villages Care Packages are focused on residents of retirement villages who require additional aged-care services to assist in their choice to stay at home for as long as possible.

Apart from government programs, private aged-care services can provide help from two hours up to twenty-four hours a day, providing a broad range of services such as respite care; personal hygiene and domestic assistance; shopping and meal preparation; medication assistance; transport, companionship, and socialization; and nursing and palliative care.

IN MANY COUNTRIES THESE SERVICES ARE NOT PROVIDED.

If people can afford this kind of service, it enables people to live comfortably at home for longer and relieves the family of much of the burden and avoids early entry into a nursing home.

Private-supported residential accommodation in a retirement village, for example, can be a feasible option if assets can be sold to pay for the unit. This arrangement can be very suitable for elderly couples, where a spouse can be supported to care for their husband or wife and yet be afforded a measure of independence and dignity.

In many countries these services are not provided. However, with the level of support provided in Australia, even these strategies are eventually not enough, especially when physical illness, reduced mobility, or failing health makes caring all that more difficult.

Entry into a nursing home or full-time in-home nursing care become the remaining choices, and cost can be a major problem. For low-income people in Australia, government-funded hostel or nursing home accommodation is available.

> MANY ARE ABLE TO CARE FOR THEMSELVES WITH
> MINIMAL SUPPORT.

Private nursing homes require a bond amounting to several thousand dollars, meaning that the family home must be sold to fund this, and even then the day-to-day costs of care can be onerous.

A novel solution may be the establishment of day-care centers for aged people with dementia, providing programs designed to improve symptoms and functioning. The idea would be to make available to families the choice of having their parents or partners who suffer from dementia, including Alzheimer's disease, cared for in day-care centers while the caregiver is at work or involved in other activities, rather than having to place them in full-time residential care.

The concept would be to provide high-quality care of people with dementia during the day to enhance health outcomes for those who suffer from Alzheimer's and other forms of dementia through the provision of well-developed and targeted programs and to alleviate much of the stress of caregivers.

FAMILIES OVER TIME FIND IT MORE AND MORE DIFFICULT

This type of facility should appeal to to care for their parents or partners, who are often relatively physically well but whose safety is jeopardized without adequate supervision.

It is thought that aged day-care centers would be a short-term solution for some 50,000 people in Australia who are worried about their future care or who are currently employing people to provide in-home care. While there are some 300,600 people with dementia (1,130,000 by 2050), there are many who are able to care for themselves or with minimal support from relatives with no formal care (85,000) or who receive some level of community care, mainly in-home services (52,000), and many in advanced stages who are in residential care (90,000), often with significant health problems.

The benefits to the community and to families of providing day-care centers could be a superior solution than have been attained under traditional residential programs, with much improved outcomes for dementia patients who otherwise might be separated from families, often prematurely, with great distress on both sides.

THERE IS CONCERN ABOUT THE COST OF HEALTH CARE.

There is growing concern about the burgeoning cost of health care and more emphasis on self-managed or community-managed care.

The gap between informal care at home (with some caregiver allowances from the Commonwealth government) and residential care is taken up to some extent by in-home support, and a lot of this is privately funded or else there is a large use of volunteers doing this work. In Australia it is estimated that to replace family caregivers with paid caregivers would cost $5.5b annually.

The concept of keeping people in their home environments and yet allowing them a safe place to stay while caregivers are at work or involved in other activities fits well with this idea. It could be a more cost-effective model compared to in-home care, often for domestic services, or more practical than intermittent respite care.

At present there are few guidelines or best-practice protocols in place for aged day-care centers. There is inadequate training and an inability to care for those who have health problems in the few day-care centers that are operating.

DAY-CARE CENTERS PROVIDE A NEW MODEL OF CARE.

Day-care centers would need to train people and to develop a new model of care to manage people with dementia, to develop programs that are known to slow the pace of dementia, and to teach people to use strategies to maximize their independence and safety.

Additionally the centers would offer psychological support and courses for caregivers and families to help them deal with their own very significant psychological issues that arise from having to care for someone with dementia. It is often like a prolonged grieving process and is isolating and confusing, resulting in depression and high levels of anxiety. One of the biggest gaps identified is the provision of services for those with dementia who also suffer from mental health problems, often unresolved grief following the death of a partner.

The aim of the program would be to provide assessment, management, and treatment for individuals with dementia, in particular Alzheimer's disease, and those with comorbid psychological and social problems associated with the disease that preserve their rights and dignity. It would also educate and inform their families about the nature of the disease and provide support services for them to deal with their own psychological issues arising from the caring of their parents or partners who have the disease by providing timely and individualized treatment.

MANY CAN CARE WITH MINIMAL SUPPORT.

The idea is to develop programs that are multi-tiered depending on thorough assessments (in addition to aged-care assessment teams streaming for government funding according to need), transitioning people from low- to high-intensity care, providing programs that are mostly self-managed with early-stage dementia through to programs providing counseling and structured activities designed to improve quality of life and meeting the expectations of families for middle- to late-stage dementia.

The aged day-care centers could provide services for a selected group of dementia patients who have developed a range of symptoms that require constant supervision, although varying levels of direct support, and who have been successfully cared for in their homes by relatives, sometimes with home care support, who find that their employment, care of other family members, and leisure time are now severely compromised and who have the potential to benefit from and could afford a day-care program as proposed.

CAREGIVERS FIND TIME IS SEVERELY COMPROMISED.

While there are some day-care centers (called respite centers) funded under the Commonwealth Respite and Carelink Centres program, there are, some large gaps in the provision of services, especially as there are few guidelines for staff ratios or training and program development. There is predicted to be a huge increase in the numbers of people with Alzheimer's and dementia and predictions of a massive shortage of trained staff to deal with the problem. There is a demand for this type of program that has not been met as yet, as there is a strong desire on behalf of patients and families to delay as long as possible people going into residential care and estimates of losses of $900m in wages due to time taken caring for this group.

The idea of developing aged day-care centers taps into an area of need that has not been available previously on a broad scale. It could be seen as a transition program between home care and full-time residential care, where the ratio of staff to patients in both in-home and residential care is approximately 1:1, compared to ratios of 1:5 to 1:10 in the aged day-care centers.

DAY-CARE CENTERS CAN SUPPORT CAREGIVERS.

Integral to the program is an assessment process that considers the biopsychosocial aspects of the disease to determine the level of care required. Dementia patients may enter the program with very few if any health or mobility problems and, therefore, require minimal supervision and can participate in a range of supervised activities that are often self-directed by the patients. On the other hand, middle- to late-stage dementia can involve significant levels of health care and close supervision as well as very challenging behavior that can be taxing on health workers.

Assessments need to determine the intensity of care and staff ratios and training that are adequate to provide this care. Staff would be allocated according to the level of care required, or else a recommendation that patients are admitted into residential care.

However, there comes a time when this type of program is no longer feasible as the person's condition deteriorates and the level of care required becomes difficult to provide in the community. The decision of when a person should move into a residential care facility must be addressed at sometime and preferably before the burden tends to overwhelm everyone, especially when you feel close to breaking down due to the constant demands, your inability to physically provide support, and when the interests of other family members are being compromised too much.

FINALLY HER MOTHER WAS ADMITTED INTO A HOME.

Indications that the time has come may include double incontinence, onset of other serious illnesses, an inability to get out of bed, aggressive or inappropriate behavior, wandering, and getting lost. Hopefully this has been discussed well before this is needed with the person with dementia and the wider family so that everyone can come to terms with the idea and prepare for this eventuality. It is sometimes difficult after you have managed to care for your loved one for some time to let go and not to feel a sense of defeat and guilt and even a sense that others will judge you harshly for abandoning your responsibility.

I spent some time counseling a woman from Greek background, who had been caring for her mother for seven years. This involved getting up very early, driving an hour to her mother's house, helping her shower, get dressed, and have breakfast while a paid caregiver sat with her during the day. She would then work all day in a demanding role as a trainer and then drive to her mother's, see she ate her dinner, and then prepare her for bed. She would finally arrive home at after eight each evening.

> PEOPLE DELAY ADMISSION UNTIL THE TOLL IS TOO HIGH.

When she came to see me, she felt that she was stressed and anxious, her marriage was deteriorating, and she had delayed having a child and feared she was now getting too old. She also felt angry that her husband, while tolerant, had not been supportive enough and that her two older brothers had left the burden to her. Of greatest concern was that she had finally allowed her mother to be admitted to a nursing home. She was racked with guilt, as she had promised her mother she would never do this to her. She was also suffering from exhaustion and grief at the loss of her mother as her mentor and friend. It took some weeks of working with her and then with her and her husband for her to find some resolution.

The types of services and facilities to someone like my client's mother are determined by an aged-care assessment team and will result in accommodation being provided in either a low- or high-level care facility. Depending on income and assets, fees will vary for daily care and accommodation.

RECENTLY NEW MODELS OF CARE HAVE EVOLVED.

Admission to high-care facilities may not require any accommodation bond. The government is presently reviewing the provision of care, and major and fundamental reforms will no doubt come in time. Focus will be on ensuring access to services by everyone needing them, more choice, including specialist services for those with dementia, and a smoother transition between types of care. We can be assured that with the rising numbers of older people who will need care, this will increasingly need to be funded by users.

It is important to look at the range of options available, affordability, and that any facility is capable of meeting the needs of someone with dementia. Many issues need to be considered, such as staff attitudes, privacy and comfort, levels of support, visitor comfort and amenities, acceptance of your suggestions, access to doctors and records, going on outings, accessibility to medical and specialist care, emergency arrangements, and a full understanding of any fees or charges.

Recently new models of care have evolved. A range of interventions developed within disabilities services have been adapted to provide innovative programs for people with dementia. The levels of advocacy for people with a range of disabilities have resulted in an awareness of the rights of this group, and the rights of those with dementia, especially younger age-onset dementia, are now starting to be recognized. No longer is it good enough for people to be shuffled off to nursing homes to be forgotten.

> THE AIM IS TO RESPECT THEM AND IMPROVE QUALITY OF LIFE.

Other models of care for people with varying stages of dementia emphasize community links, such as the Intergenerational Learning projects in the United States and independent living that involves the establishment of small group homes in local communities. The aim is to respect their dignity and to improve the quality of life for these people.

The next chapter raises the issue of quality of life for the person with dementia. It is one thing to have lived a long life, reaping the benefits of a wealthy economy and privileged existence. It is quite another matter to consider the possibility of living well with the disease.

Chapter 13

Quality of Life and Living with Dementia

Quality of life is a very difficult subject to deal with, as it contains many complexities that are both practical, historical, social, and moral. For someone with dementia, quality of life and dementia seem mutually exclusive. It is a feared, disabling, alienating, and terminal disease. For later stage dementia, quality of life can be complicated by illness and sensory loss that can limit functioning.

FOCUS NEEDS TO SHIFT TO THE PERSON WITH DEMENTIA.

However, an environment that optimizes quality of life for those who have dementia is unmistakable when it is encountered. Anyone who has spent time in aged-care facilities knows they can be the saddest and most dispiriting places or they can be the "happiest ward in the hospital."

Moreover, quality of life for people with dementia has not been the focus of widespread attention until recently. Services have tended to have the welfare of the caregiver as the driving force in the provision of services. Aged-care facilities are about taking over when caregivers can't cope, or where there is no caregiver and the community can't deal with someone who can no longer look after themselves; day care is called respite care, and it is the caregiver who is being catered to. In this process some programs enhance the quality of life, but they have done this almost as a side thought. Nursing homes are about minding people when no one else can or will; day-care programs are about keeping someone safe while the caregiver has, needless to say, given the burden of caring day in, day out, a well-earned break.

> **THE AIM IS TO IMPROVE THE QUALITY FOR BOTH CARE AND CARED FOR.**

Palliative care in the latter stages of life is concerned with quality of life, or at least minimizing suffering, whereas the care provided to the person with dementia should also have quality of life as the primary focus. This is now being acknowledged and programs designed for the patient's, rather than anyone else's, needs.

While the needs of the caregiver are important, the focus needs to shift to programs primarily concerned with the needs of the person with dementia to improve the quality of life. The goal must be not just freedom from pain or material well-being, but lives full of joy and fulfillment. As a result the needs of caregivers will also be addressed. Good quality of life can be achieved encouraging caregivers to be more engaged and involved in the care of their elderly relatives. A sad, despondent atmosphere will not encourage involvement by caregivers, once their loved one is secure in a residential facility. It seems that very few relatives ever or regularly visit their loved ones in aged-care facilities.

The pall of loneliness that can only be partly replaced by staff attentiveness. When a regular visitor arrives there is a change in mood. The smiles, the laughter, the talk increase noticeably. The sad thing is that the visitor is often not their relative, but someone else's. However, this is one of the few friendly faces they will see as they wait hour after hour, day after day for someone to come to see them.

QUALITY OF LIFE FOR THE PERSON WITH DEMENTIA IS RELATED TO HIGHER QUALITY OF LIFE FOR CAREGIVERS

An aged-care facility or day-care program that enhances the quality of life, that lifts moods and replaces sadness and inertia with joy and fun, can improve functioning as a side effect of enhanced mood. That benefits everyone, including caregivers, as studies have shown that improved quality of life for caregivers is related to higher quality of life for the person with dementia. The greater the burden and the poorer quality of life for caregivers, the lower the quality of life is for the dementia sufferer.

What do we mean by quality of life and how do we define it? What does quality of life mean for someone who can't communicate as they have lost the use of language or who can't remember what they did that morning? How do we measure it, and how do we know if we are making a difference?

QUALITY OF LIFE AND DEPRESSION ARE HIGHLY RELATED.

What have we found? For people with dementia, quality of life is not a function of age. Level of education has not been found to be associated with quality of life. There is no difference in measures of quality of life between men and women who suffer dementia. Insight does not predict quality of life, and level of cognitive function or dementia severity does not predict differences in quality of life.

The strongest association that has been consistently found is between levels of depression and quality of life. However, caregiver quality of life is strongly associated with the quality of life of the person with dementia, and the higher the quality of life of the sufferer, the higher the quality of life of the caregiver.

As mentioned above, we know when we walk into a place whether the residents are happy and engaged or not, and we equate this with quality of life. However, if we want to be more scientific, the problem becomes more complicated. However, it seems impossible to come to any agreement as research into quality of life has been marked by competing concepts, definitions, measures, models, and theories.

ANXIETY CAN AFFECT QUALITY OF LIFE.

Despite this lack of agreement, psychologists have devised a number of instruments to measure health-related quality of life, and these have been applied to those with dementia. An obvious place to begin is to measure symptoms thought to relate to depression. Certainly quality of life and levels of depression are highly associated.

Studies have shown that in 30 to 40 percent of cases, depression is associated with poor performance on cognitive tests, and it is associated with increased risk of dementia. However, it is clear that in a majority of cases, depression coincides with or follows the onset of symptoms, rather than precedes it.

So, depression may be a cause of dementia, or it may be symptom of dementia, or is it that people's needs are neglected? Often apathy is documented as a symptom of dementia. In one group of residents, 13 percent showed signs of depression, whereas 64 percent showed signs of apathy.

Is apathy then a sign of depression or a separately measured entity? None of this is clear, but at least a part of the depression is due to life circumstances: lack of love and nurturing, loss of loved ones and friends, loss of functioning and loss of role, loss of hope, abandonment, and dealing with the reality of a terminal disease. And so it can be treated in much the same way psychologists treat other forms of reactive depression.

> APATHY MAY BE A SIGN OF DEPRESSION.

But is treating depression the same as improving quality of life? Are we measuring and improving quality of life (perhaps equated with depressed mood) or treating health issues (depressive disorder)? Use of cognitive behavioral therapy (CBT) and long-term use of antidepressants in the treatment of late-life depression have not been particularly successful.

However, treating depression is not the only way we improve the quality of life and the effectiveness of treatment. Indeed, levels of anxiety can reflect on perceived quality of life. Late-life anxiety and apathy could be associated with changes in neurological pathways.

Behavioral and psychological disturbance have been associated with poorer quality of life for caregivers. To deal with difficult behavior, it has been reported that some 30 percent and up to 87 percent of nursing home residents are medicated using antipsychotics, Antipsychotics have been shown to reduce hallucinations and aggression. However, not only are some dementias made worse by these drugs; overuse of this medication as a patient management tool could be seen as abusive. On the other hand, studies have shown that changes toward person-centered care and to the environment lead to a reduction of behavioral and psychological problems more effectively than these drugs.

A CARING ENVIRONMENT INCLUDES A FLEXIBLE ROUTINE.

Simple changes in routine events such as bathing, dressing and feeding have been shown to reduce agitation, aggression, and discomfort, while use of more involved interventions such as multisensory-stimulation rooms and childhood memory boxes have shown improvements in agitation, aggression, mood, and apathy. A person-centered caring environment includes a flexible approach to routine events, taking time to find out what someone wants or needs to do and responding empathically, providing a stimulating program of activities, such as dance, song, and play, and not enforcing engagement or change as it may not be wanted.

Quality of life is the ability to make choices from a range of options. This implies two things. First is that a range of choices is not limited and not imposed: who provides the choices and who does the choosing? The reality is the quality of life of the caregiver takes priority and the range and capacity for choice is limited by the needs of the caregiver. Even when choices are available, the older person may not want to change. They may deliberately choose to reduce their level of activity in order to continue with a smaller range of activities they value.

HOW DO WE KNOW WHAT IS EFFECTIVE?

Second it implies that the person with dementia can make meaningful decisions about the choices offered. However, among people with dementia, cognitive decline may detract from their capacity for discernment and their ability to make choices that maximize benefit. For example, their ability to delay gratification to achieve much better longer-term outcomes. Often in later stages, the capacity to articulate, let alone being able to meaningfully make choices can be severely compromised.

So, what is important and how do we know what to do and what we are doing is effective? No matter how well-meaning, it is very much subjective.

We could ask the same questions of the care of our newborn babies, where similarly, language in a meaningful sense is not the medium, and memory, apart from the occasional smile of recognition, is not a component.

DEMENTIA IS ALL TOO REAL FOR MANY FAMILIES.

What we do is provide lots of attention, touching, smiling, pointless chitchat, cuddles, holding, and just being close by. And how do we know it's working? It's the body language, the smiles and giggles, the look of contentment; peaceful sleep and interested wakefulness. In the case of a child, we don't speak of treatment to improve the quality of life. We take it for granted that our role is to ensure the best possible life for our growing babies. Why do we not think of our elderly in the same way?

Despite our best efforts, the reality of dementia is all too real for many families. Overcoming and dealing with these difficulties can be very challenging.

The next chapter of this book looks at legal issues that may affect people with dementia or their families and how these issues may be managed to protect the rights of everyone involved. Again I try to focus on practical solutions to deal with difficult and painful problems as the disease progresses and mental processes become more impaired.

Chapter 14

Legal Issues: Talk about It While You Can

People with dementia inevitably get to a stage where their ability to make decisions for themselves is severely impaired. These decisions can relate to a range of matters, such as health care, living situation, their finances, property, and legal action. They can be dealt with in different ways, from informal arrangements involving you and your family making decisions to a range of formal legal processes.

> YOUR WISHES CAN BE CLEAR IN A LEGAL DOCUMENT.

The question arises as to when it is appropriate or necessary to seek legal protection, either by placing affairs in the hands of a trusted relative or the hands of someone appointed by the state. For the person who has dementia in its early stages, the answer is simple. Either make arrangements now, or wait until it is taken out of their hands.

In the case of a will, which is legally binding, it should be high on the agenda of anyone who reaches their later years as they have the choice of who they appoint as executor and who they trust to carry out their instructions. The role of the executor is to proceed according to their instructions to the extent they accord with the applicable laws. The same principle should also apply when the person with dementia is still able to make sound decisions regarding their daily affairs while they are alive. A lawyer can help determine who the best person is to carry out instructions, and this can be made clear in a properly executed legal document. Again, these instructions need to accord with the law and also be a realistic appraisal of the person's financial position, as well as their perceived needs and best interests.

LEGAL ARRANGEMENTS PROTECT THE RIGHTS OF PEOPLE.

The drawing up of an advanced-care directive can be helpful, although not legally binding. Among other things, this document can be useful to introduce yourself as an individual. It can be useful for medical teams to be able to treat a person who cannot speak for themselves if health takes a substantial turn for the worse. It can make clear in what circumstances you would consider it unacceptable to artificially extend life and provide instructions for treatment if there is no reasonable chance of recovery.

Many countries have legal models designed to protect the rights of people who lose the capacity to make decisions and to care for themselves, although the processes and mechanics vary considerably. It is important to seek specific advice from the country or state authorities where you live.

To provide an example, I will describe the system that is in place in New South Wales, where I lived. To do so I have extracted information from the NSW government website: www.publicguardian.justice.nsw.gov.au. More detailed information can be found on this website: see page 185.

see page 185.

> ## ENDURING GUARDIANS DO NOT MAKE FINANCIAL DECISIONS.

The person you care about can prepare for the time when they are unable to make good decisions by having a guardian appointed under an enduring guardianship arrangement. The appointment is a legal agreement, where someone is nominated by them to make health and welfare decisions, for example, where they live and the health care they receive. "Enduring" means the arrangement continues (endures) when they are unable to make these types of decisions. The enduring guardian can start making decisions when the person loses the capacity to do so and have the same legal force as a guardian appointed by the Guardianship Tribunal.

An enduring guardian can only consent to medical and dental treatment that will promote or maintain health and well-being. However, they cannot make or alter a will, they cannot vote or consent to marriage. Where the person with dementia objects to treatment or special medical treatment they cannot consent to that medical or dental treatment.

EUTHANASIA IS ILLEGAL.

Only after particular discussion can the Guardianship Tribunal can this authority be given. Also, they cannot make decisions that are against the law, like euthanasia or breaking a legally binding contract.

Enduring guardians cannot make financial decisions unless they have also been appointed as a financial manager or enduring power of attorney as well, but these are different roles.

Binding directions can be made when appointing an enduring guardian. The person with dementia can direct the guardian to make decisions that when the directions are made as part of the witnessed appointment, are relevant to the decision that needs to be made, and the person is competent to make those directions.

If there are concerns about your loved one's welfare and well-being under an enduring guardianship form of appointment, anyone with a genuine concern, including you and your family, can apply to the Guardianship Tribunal to review the appointment. The tribunal can then review the situation, and any appointment made at a hearing and based on the findings may then be upheld, varied, revoked, or suspended, or the tribunal may make a guardianship order.

WHO IS RESPONSIBLE FOR DECISIONS THAT AFFECT YOU?

Enduring guardianship ends when the person dies or the guardian resigns, or the appointment is revoked by the person who made the appointment (while they have capacity), the Guardianship Tribunal, or the Supreme Court.

Enduring guardianship appointments set are only valid in New South Wales, and if the person with dementia moves to another state or territory, the guardian would need to seek recognition of their appointment from the equivalent guardianship tribunal body in the new state or territory.

The question may arise as to wishes regarding the prolonging of the life of the person with dementia when they might express the view that they might be better off to be allowed to depart this earth gracefully. At this time euthanasia is illegal, and it would be impossible for someone to claim they were carrying out the will of your loved one to end their life under normal circumstances, but especially if advanced dementia has taken hold. No one would suggest that they had any competence to make such a decision, and any suggestion they did, especially if someone else stood to benefit, would be wrong.

> ## A PERSON WITH LEGAL AUTHORITY CAN MAKE DECISIONS FOR THE PERSON WITH DEMENTIA.

This same issue of competency would also be relevant if the person with dementia were to write a will or make some other decision that might impact on others when they have reached a state where judgment can be determined to be unreliable. Evidence would no doubt be required to satisfy a court that they did have the capacity to make such decisions. In some cases legal authorities could appoint someone to make these decisions for them.

In the event that the person with dementia has not made these decisions, then relatives who are the caregivers, but who might also stand to benefit, have the difficult task of deciding when and if the time has arrived to seek legal advice and then to make decisions that fundamentally affect your spouse's or father's or mother's life and, in turn, your life. It is possible that any decision made could be challenged, and a legal representative should be involved.

Under the Guardianship Act 1987 (NSW), a person can be appointed to make decisions on behalf of the person with dementia.

LEGAL GUARDIANS CAN MAKE HEALTH DECISIONS.

However, only if it is considered that they lack decision-making capacity concerning personal and life choices because of dementia or other disability, except decisions about financial matters or the person's estate unless they have been appointed as the person's financial manager under an enduring power of attorney or have been appointed by the Guardianship Tribunal, the Mental Health Review Tribunal, or the Supreme Court.

In a recent case, a woman sought my advice regarding her mother, who was well into her eighties and spoke no English and who was showing signs of forgetfulness and confusion about where she lived, applied to the tribunal to take control of her mother's affairs based on the advice of her mother's doctor and due to her own concerns, especially about the amount of money her mother was giving to her overbearing older sister. In this case the tribunal refused the application because her mother did not agree to the order and they considered her to be competent. She reported that, as a result, her mother had become distant and accused her of wanting to steal her money. This behavior was very hurtful as she visited her mother daily and took her to do all her shopping and on outings and to her doctor's appointments, whereas other relatives, including the sister, hardly ever visited or helped.

> **ADULTS ARE ASSUMED TO BE COMPETENT TO MAKE DECISIONS.**

A year later the same woman came to me complaining that the sister had arranged to have the rent on a property the mother owned paid to her instead of the mother. She had convinced the tenant she had legal guardianship. Some eight months of rent had gone before my client realized what had occurred, as her mother had not noticed the missing amounts. As the property was in Turkey, I thought that the chances of recovering the lost money would be very difficult, but that in view of this, she should again approach the tribunal to have the decision changed. Despite what had happened, she was reluctant to do so as she feared her mother's reaction as it had caused so much distress for her before.

In a case such as this or when there is no suitable private person who can be appointed guardian, the tribunal can appoint the public guardian to make decisions for them if they believe there is sufficient evidence to support this decision.

When there are issues regarding health or living situation, legal guardians can be appointed, whereas matters relating to financial or legal matters require the appointment of a legal administrator, such as a public trustee.

RELATIVES ARE LEFT MAKE DAY-TO-DAY DECISIONS

It is usually assumed at law that all adults over the age of eighteen have the capacity and competence to make decisions regarding their welfare and the management of their affairs, unless it can be shown that dementia or some other disease or injury is affecting their decision-making ability. In this case it is necessary that someone else should make these decisions, but the decisions of that person can be open to challenge if decisions supposedly made in the best interests of the person with dementia are questionable.

Of course in the ordinary course of things, if the person with dementia does not appear to object or dispute a decision, then it is reasonable and acceptable that relatives and caregivers make day-to-day decisions regarding most matters on the person's behalf. If there appears to be agreement among the parties, it is reasonable for third parties to assume that consent by the person with dementia has been given. If, however, the consequences of any decision are drastic or irreversible, then these informal arrangements may come under scrutiny, even if the person with dementia does not voice objection.

A POWER OF ATTORNEY MANAGES FINANCIAL AFFAIRS.

As in the case related above and in similar circumstances, arrangements are made to appoint an outside legal guardian to protect the rights of the person with dementia. These situations may arise when there is a dispute about what is appropriate care between caregivers and health professionals, where treatment is risky or ethically contentious or involves special procedures, or where legal consent is required by law.

Each country and state has different legislation to regulate decision making on behalf of people with dementia and other disabilities and the appointment of legal guardians.

In New South Wales, the provision of services is entrusted to the NSW Trustee and Guardian. This service is legally constituted to provide professional and independent trustee services, making of wills, acting as executor in the deceased's estates, and managing trusts and power of attorney. Again I have extracted information from the NSW government website: http://www.tag.nsw.gov.au/what-is-a-power-of-attorney.html.

> # A POWER OF ATTORNEY IS AS IMPORTANT AS MAKING A WILL.

Many people prepare a will but neglect to appoint an attorney until it is too late. A power of attorney can be as necessary for life planning as making a will. Appointing someone to act in this role gives them the legal authority to look after financial affairs on behalf of the person with dementia.

When they are no longer able to manage their affairs a person can appoint an attorney to act for them. NSW Trustee and Guardian (formerly Public Trustee NSW) can act as attorney and can help identify the type of attorney service that suits the person's needs so people with dementia can be confident of having an independent, impartial, and skilled asset manager to manage their financial affairs.

Power of attorney offers three levels of planned assistance: a power of attorney designed to provide a safety net should unforeseen events occur, such as worsening of symptoms of the disease; a safe account to secure savings; and a power of attorney where the person can choose the level of assistance he or she requires. These three levels enable the attorney to manage financial affairs when the person is not competent to make those decisions.

THE PERSON WITH DEMENTIA WANTS TO CONTROL THIER AFFAIRS

The reasons for appointing using a power of attorney may be that people with dementia do not wish to burden their families or friends with the responsibility of looking after their financial affairs, or it may be they find the demands of financial management have become too much for them to handle. The person with dementia may wish to be free of the day-to-day demands of financial paperwork and record keeping, and he or she may want to place funds in a secure, government guaranteed account that attracts interest and flexible access.

Both caregivers and those with dementia are entitled to a range of benefits. These include a caregiver's allowance, a caregiver payment, which is subject to income and asset tests, pharmaceutical allowances, rent assistance, telephone allowance, bereavement payment and in-home support. A pensioner concession card will facilitate many of these benefits, such as reduced rates, power bills, ambulance services, and car registration. Contacting Centrelink and Aged Care Australia will provide information about how these benefits and concessions can be accessed.

DO NOT BE AFRAID TO ASK.

The vital issue is that the person with dementia would want to control his or her affairs for as long as possible. When this is not feasible anymore, we need to know where to find help. The following resource section has some contact details to make finding help somewhat easier. Do not be afraid to ask.

Resources

Access to Community Care: 1800 052 222 (business hours).
For emergency respite support outside standard business
hours: 1800 059.

Advanced Care Directive. Dr. Lyndon Bauer,
lyndon@healthpromotion.com.au.

Aged Care Australia: www.agedcareaustralia.gov.au.
A government department that seeks to promote, develop,
and fund health and aged-care services for the Australian
public.

Aged Care Information Line: 1800 500 853.

Ageing Well: www.ageingwell.org.au.
Aging well is about emotional well-being, as well as good
mental and physical function. Socializing and participating in
physical activity and eating healthy foods are good for both
your emotional and physical health.

Alzheimer's Australia: www.alzheimers.org.au. The peak
body providing support and advocacy for people living with

dementia. Includes sections on services, support, education, training, and a help line.

Australian Psychological Society Referral Line: 1800 333497.

Carers NSW: www.carersnsw.asn.au.
Carers NSW is an association for relatives and friends caring for people with a disability, mental illness, drug and alcohol dependencies, chronic condition, or terminal illness, or who are frail.

Centrelink: 132717.

Commonwealth Carer Resource Centre: 1800 100 500.

Dementia Care Australia (DCA):
www.dementiacareaustralia.com.
Dementia Care Australia (DCA) is an independent information and education organization specializing in supporting both people with dementia and their caregivers, be they family members, professional caregivers, employers, or friends.

Diabetes Australia: 1300 136588.
www.diabetesaustralia.com.au. Information about diabetes.

Grief Link. Website: www.grieflink.asn.au/aboutgrief.html.

Self-testing website: www.mindcheck.com.au. E-mail:
ross@addictiontreatment.com.au.

National Continence Helpline: 1800 033 066.

National Heart Foundation: 1300 362787.
www.heartfoundation.com.au.
Information on heart health.

NSW Trustee and Guardian: 1300 364 103. Website:
www.tag.nsw.gov.au/.
19 O'Connell Street, Sydney NSW 2000.
GPO Box 7, Sydney NSW 2001.
Ph: (02) 9252 0523; Fx: (02) 9231 4527.
Private Guardian Support Unit (PGSU): 02 8688 6060; e-
mail: informationsupport@opg.nsw.gov.au.

Respite Services: 1800 052 222 (business hours). For
emergency respite support outside standard business hours:
1800 059 059.

Acknowledgments

I would like express my gratitude to David Hammer and Martin Costanzo, who have inspired and helped me to complete this book. Leon Fink has been extraordinary in his generous support. I would also like to thank Shelley Li, who has patiently supported my efforts to write a book that she also believes will be of benefit to those who are struggling with the burden of dementia. I also owe a debt of thanks for those who worked in the clinic and supported my work and those who read the book and who made helpful suggestions: Annie Li, Lyne De Salis, Dr Penny Brabin, Dr Barry Landa, Dr David Hunt, Dr David Jansen, Michael Manuel, Tom Greally, Chris Ozsywa and Hon Kay Hull. Lastly I would like to thank all those I have worked with who have been affected by dementia and by alcoholism and brain injury; I have witnessed amazing courage and compassion over the years.

References

Access Economics (2009). *Keeping Dementia Front of Mind: Incidence and Prevalence 2009–2050*. Alzheimer's Australia; Sydney.

Access Economics (2009). *Projections of Dementia Prevalence and Incidence in NSW*. Alzheimer's Australia; Sydney.

Alsop, D. C., Detre, J. A., & Grossman, M. (2000). Assessment of cerebral blood flow in Alzheimer's disease by spin-labeled magnetic resonance imaging. *Annals of Neurology*, Vol. 47(1), pp. 93–100. DOI: 10.1002/1531-8249(200001)47:1<93::AID-ANA15>3.0.CO;2-8.

Alzheimer's Association. Alzheimer's and diet. http://evergreencottages.com/blog/.

Alzheimer's Association. Be heart smart. http://www.alz.org/we_can_help_be_heart_smart.asp.

Alzheimer's Australia. Living with dementia. www.alzheimers.org.au.

Archer, J. (1999). *The Nature of Grief*. Rutledge; London.

Ashfield, J. (2008). *Taking Care of Yourself and Your Family*. Peacock; Adelaide.

Australian and New Zealand College of Anaesthetists and Faculty of Pain Management (2010). Acute Pain Management: Scientific Evidence. P. E. Macintyre, D. A. Scott, S. A. Schug, E. J. Visor, & S. M. Walker (Eds.), Australian and New Zealand College of Anaesthetists; Melbourne.

Bartenstein, P., Minoshima, S., Hirsch, C., Buch, K., Willoch, F., Mösch, D. & Kurz, A. (1997). Quantitative assessment of cerebral blood flow in patients with Alzheimer's disease by SPECT. *Journal of Nuclear Medicine: Official Publication, Society of Nuclear Medicine*, Vol. 38(7), pp. 1095–1101.

Bartholomew, A. (2012). *The Truth about Vitamins and Minerals: Choosing the Nutrients You Need to Stay Healthy.* Harvard University Press: Boston.

Bell, R. D., & Zlokovic, B. V. (2009). Neurovascular mechanisms and blood–brain barrier disorder in Alzheimer's disease. *Acta Neuropathologica*, Vol. 118(1), pp. 103–113. DOI: 10.1007/s00401-009-0522-3.

Benerjee, S., Samsi, K., Petrie, C. D., Alvir, J. Treglia, M., Schwam, E. M., & del Valle, M. What do we know about quality of life in dementia? *International Journal of Geriatric Psychiatry*, 2009, Vol. 24, pp. 15–24.

Boeve, B. F., & Boxer, A. L. (2009). Dementia treatment. In *The Behavioural Neurology of Dementia*. (B. L. Miller & B. F. Boeve, Eds.). Cambridge; New York.

Cabot, S. (2005). Alzheimer's: What you must know to protect your brain and improve your memory. WHAS; Camden, Australia.

Chan, S., Chiu, H., Chien, W-T., Goggins, W., Thompson, D., Lam, L., & Hong, B. (2009). Predicting changes in the health-related quality of life of Chinese depressed older people. *International Journal of Geriatric Psychiatry*, 2009, Vol. 24, pp. 41–47.

Chester, R., & Bender, M. (2003). *Understanding Dementia.* Jessica Kingsley; London.

Christennsen, L., & Coltrera, F. (2014). *A Guide to Coping with Alzheimer's Disease.* Harvard University Press; Boston

Cohen-Mansfield, J. (2001). Managing agitation in elderly patients with dementia. *Geriatric Times*, Vol. II (3).

Cohen-Mansfield, J., & Biling, N. (1986). Agitated behaviour in the elderly. A conceptual review. *Journal of the American Geriatric Society,* Vol. 34(10), pp. 711–721.

Cohen-Mansfield, J., Marx, M. S., & Rosenthal, A. S. (1990). Dementia and agitation in nursing home residents: How are they related? *Psychology and Aging*, Vol. 5 (1), pp. 3–8.

Cohen-Mansfield, J., & Werner, P. (1995). Environmental influences on agitation: An integrative summary of an observational study. *American Journal of Alzheimer's Disease and Other Dementias* 10(1):32–39.

Craig, A. H., Cummings, J. L., Fairbanks, L., Itti, L., Miller, B. L., Li, J., & Mena, I. (1996). Cerebral blood flow correlates of apathy in Alzheimer disease. *Archives of Neurology*, Vol. 53(11), p. 1116-1121.

Dacamay, E. Dementia: Five dietary guidelines to help manage symptoms._http://leukemia-cll.blogspot.com.au/2009/08/dementia-five-dietary-guidelines-to.html.

Dai, W., Lopez, O. L., Carmichael, O. T., Becker, J. T., Kuller, L. H., & Gach, H. M. (2009). Mild cognitive impairment and Alzheimer disease: Patterns of altered cerebral blood flow at MR imaging. *Radiology*, Vol. 250(3), p. 856-864. DOI: 10.1148/radiol.2503080751.

de la Torre, J. C. (2010). Vascular risk factor detection and control may prevent Alzheimer's disease. *Ageing Research Reviews*, Vol. 9(3), pp. 218–225.

de la Torre, J. C. (2012). A turning point for Alzheimer's disease? *Biofactors*, Vol. 38(2), pp. 78–83. DOI: 10.1002/biof.200.

Dementia Collaborative Research Centres (2009). UNSW Newsletter. www.dementia.unsw.edu.au.

Department of Health and Ageing (2006). Dementia: The caring experience. Commonwealth of Australia; Canberra. www.ag.gov.au/cca.

Department of Health and Ageing (2006). Living with dementia. Commonwealth of Australia; Canberra. www.ag.gov.au/cca.

Ettema, T. P., Droes, R. M., Lange, J. D., Mellenbergh, G. J., & Ribbe, M. W. (2007). QUALIDEM development of a dementia-specific quality of life instrument—Validation. *International Journal of Geriatric Psychiatry*, 2007, Vol. 22 (5), pp. 424–430.

Feil, N. (1993). *The Validation Breakthrough: Simple Techniques for Communicating with People with Alzheimer's-Type Dementia.* MacLennan & Petty; Sydney.

Gurland, B. J., & Gurland, R. V. (2009). The choices, choosing model of quality of life: Description and rationale. *International Journal of Geriatric Psychiatry*, 2009, Vol. 24, pp. 90–95.

Halpern, G. (2000). *Ginko: A Practical Guide*. Penguin; Australia.

Hamilton-Craig, I. (2008). *Unclog Your Arteries: Prevent Heart Attack and Stroke and Live a Longer Healthier Life*. New Holland; Sydney.

Hebben, N., & Milberg, W. (2002). *Essentials of Neuropsychological Assessment*. John Wiley; New York.

Hodges, J. R. (2007). *Cognitive Assessment for Clinicians*. Oxford; New York.

House of Representatives Standing Committee on Health and Ageing. (2013). *Thinking Ahead: Report on the Enquiry into Dementia: Early Diagnosis and Intervention*. Commonwealth of Australia; Canberra.

Humpel, C. (2011). Chronic mild cerebrovascular dysfunction as a cause for Alzheimer's disease? *Experimental Gerontology*, Vol. 46(4), 225–232. DOI: 10.1016/j.exger.2010.11.032.

Humphrey, G. M., & Zimpfer, D. G. *Counselling for Grief and Bereavement*. Sage; London.

Hungerford, C. (2006). *Good Health in the 21st Century*. Scribe; Melbourne.

Iadecola, C. (2004). Neurovascular regulation in the normal brain and in Alzheimer's disease. *Nature Reviews Neuroscience*, Vol. 5(5), pp. 347–360. DOI:10.1038/nrn1387.

Kahle-Wrobleski, K., Corrado, M. M., & Kawas, C. H. (2009). Dementia and cognition in the olderst-old. In *The Behavioural Neurology of Dementia*. (B. L. Miller & B. F. Boeve, Eds.). Cambridge; New York.

Koopmans, R. T. C. M., van der Molen, M., Raats, M., & Ettema, T. P. (2009). Neuropsychiatric symptoms and quality of life in patients in the final phase of dementia. *International Journal of Geriatric Psychiatry*, 2009, Vol. 24, pp. 25–32.

Korczyn, A. D., & Halperin, I. (2009). Depression and dementia. *Journal of the Neurological Sciences*. Vol. 283(1–2), Aug. 2009, pp. 139–142.

Larner, A. J. (2008). *Neurophysiological Neurology*. Cambridge; New York.

Lennox, N., & Diggens, J. (Eds.) (1999). *Management Guidelines for People with Developmental and Intellectual Disabilities*. Therapeutic Guidelines; Melbourne.

Lenze, E. J., & Wetherell, J. L. (2009). Bring the bedside to the bench and then to the community: A prospectus for intervention research in late-life anxiety disorders. *International Journal of Geriatric Psychiatry*, 2009, Vol. 24, pp. 1–14.

Lewis, M., & Lewis, G. (2007). *Dietary Supplements: Creating Expensive Urine or a key to Modern Medicine?* Lewins Publications; Auckland, NZ.

Li Yubin (2015). Revealing the Mystery of Traditional Chinese Medicine: A Practical Guide to Curing Diseases. Editors. Jian Huifang and Ross Colquhoun. In press

Liddel, B. J., Paul, R. H., Arns, M., Gordon, N., Kukla, M., & Rowe, D. (2007). Rates of decline distinguish Alzheimer's disease and mild cognitive impairment relative to normal aging: Integrating cognition and brain function. *Journal of Integrative Neuroscience*, Vol. 6 (1), pp. 141–174.

Liebling, A., & Cohen, L. (2006). *Thinking about Dementia.* Rutgers University Press; New Brunswick, NH, USA

Lifestyle factors and risk of dementia.

http://www.mja.com.au/public/issues/184_02_160106/sim1 0682_fm.html.

Matsuda, H. (2001). Cerebral blood flow and metabolic abnormalities in Alzheimer's disease. *Annals of Nuclear Medicine*, Vol. 15(2), 85–92. DOI: 10.1007/BF02988596.

Miller, B. L., & Boeve, B. F., Eds. (2009). *The Behavioural Neurology of Dementia*. Cambridge; New York.

Miller, E. A., Schneider, L. S., & Rosenheck, R. A. (2009). Assessing the relationship between health utilities, quality of life and health services use in Alzheimer's disease. *International Journal of Geriatric Psychiatry*, 2009, Vol. 24, pp. 96–105.

Namazi, K. H., & Johnson, B. D. (1992). Pertinent autonomy for residents with dementias: Modification of the physical environment to enhance independence. *American Journal of Alzheimer's Disease and Related Disorders and Research*, Vol. 7(1), pp. 16–21.

Osiecki, H. *The Nutrient Bible, 9th Edition*. Bio Concepts; Eagle Farm, QLD.

Ponsford, J. (2002). *Traumatic Brain Injury: Rehabilitation for Everyday Adaptive Living*. Psychology Press: East Sussex.

Productivity Commission (2010). Caring for older Australians: A public inquiry into Australia's aged care arrangements. www.pc.gov.au/projects/inquiry/aged-care.

Scarmeas, N., Zarahn, E., Anderson, K. E., Habeck, C. G., Hilton, J., Flynn, J. & Stern, Y. (2003). Association of life activities with cerebral blood flow in Alzheimer disease: Implications for the cognitive reserve hypothesis. *Archives of Neurology*, Vol. 60(3), pp. 359–365. DOI:10.1001/archneur.60.3.359.

Schauss, A. G. (2009). *Acai from the Amazon.* Biosocial; Tacoma, WA, USA.

Smith, M. A., & Perry, G. (1995). Free radical damage, iron and Alzheimer's disease. *New England Journal of Medicine*, Vol. 134, pp. 92–94.

Starkstein, S. E., Sabe, L., Vázquez, S., Tesón, A., Petracca, G., Chemerinski, E. & Leiguarda, R. (1996). Neuropsychological, psychiatric, and cerebral blood flow findings in vascular dementia and Alzheimer's disease. *Stroke,* 27(3), 408–414.

Strand, R. D. (2009). *Bionutrition*. Health Concepts Publishing: Rapid City, SD, USA.

Strand, R. D., & Wallace, D. K. (2002). *What Your Doctor Doesn't Know about Nutritional Medicine.* Ray Strand Publishing; Erina, NSW.

US Department of Health and Human Services. (2009). Screening for dementia. www.ahrq.gov/clinic/3rduspstf/dementia.

Venneri, A., Shanks, M. F., Staff, R. T., Pestell, S. J., Forbes, K. E., Gemmell, H. G., & Murray, A. D. (2002). Cerebral blood flow and cognitive responses to rivastigmine treatment in Alzheimer's disease. *Neuroreport*, Vol. 13(1), pp. 83–87.

Weil, A., Fox, S., & Stebner, M. (2012). *True Food: Seasonal, Sustainable, Simple, Pure.* Little, Brown & Co.; New York.

Wentz, M. (2004). *Invisible Miracles: The Revolution in Cellular Nutrition.* Medicis; South Carolina, USA.

Wilkinson, P., Adler, N., Juszczak, E., Matthews, H.& Merritt, C. (2009). A pilot randomised controlled trial of brief cognitive behavioural group intervention to reduce recurrence rates in late life depression. *International Journal of Geriatric Psychiatry*, Vol. 24, pp. 68–75.

World Health Organisation. (2004). *Management of Mental Disorders*, Vol. 2, 4th Edition. World Health Organisation; Sydney.

Yaffe, K., & Barnes, D. E. (2009). Epidemiology and Risk factors. In *The Behavioural Neurology of Dementia.* (B. L. Miller & B. F. Boeve, Eds.). Cambridge; New York.

Zafrilla, P. (2006). Oxidative stress in Alzheimer's patients in different stages of the disease. *Current Medical Chemistry*, Vol. 13 (9), pp. 1075–83.

Index

www.ingramcontent.com/pod-product-compliance
Lightning Source LLC
Chambersburg PA
CBHW070644290526
45790CB00001B/184